Keto Made Simple

The Beginner's Guide to Embracing the Ketogenic Diet

SOPHIA RAMOS

Table of Content

Introduction...8

Chapter 1: Understanding the Ketogenic Diet...11

Chapter 2: The Science Behind Keto............26

Chapter 3: Starting Your Keto Journey...........48

Chapter 4: Essential Kitchen Setup for Keto..60

Chapter 5: Keto-Friendly Grocery Shopping...74

Chapter 6: Mastering Keto Cooking Techniques..84

Chapter 7: Delicious, Easy-to-Follow Keto Recipes..92

Chapter 8: Overcoming Common Keto Challenges...102

Chapter 9: Keto and Exercise: A Comprehensive Guide...111

Chapter 10: Keto for the Long Haul: Sustainability and Adaptation..121

Chapter 11: Your Keto Lifestyle: Tips and Tricks for Success..135

Closing Remarks...............................147

Sophia Ramos

Introduction:

The ketogenic diet, more commonly known as 'keto', has been gathering fame and followers over the years due to its potential health benefits and ability to aid in weight loss. This diet is based on a high-fat, low-carbohydrate, dietary plan designed to put your body into a metabolic state known as 'ketosis'. It's a revolutionary approach to eating!.

The Ketogenic Diet Book for Beginners

Chapter 1, "Understanding the Ketogenic Diet," demystifies the concept of the ketogenic diet and provides a basic overview of what it entails and the fundamental principles behind it.

In Chapter 2, "The Science Behind Keto," delves deeper into the science of the ketogenic diet, understanding how it works on a biochemical level, and how it impacts your body.

Chapter 3, "Starting Your Keto Journey," is all about setting the stage for your successful transition into a ketogenic lifestyle. It provides actionable advice on how to prepare mentally and physically for the change.

Chapter 4, "Essential Kitchen Setup for Keto," guides you on setting up your kitchen and selecting the right tools and equipment for creating delectable keto meals.

Chapter 5 , "Keto-Friendly Grocery Shopping," offers comprehensive guidance on how to shop for keto-friendly foods. It contains a thorough list of foods to enjoy and those to avoid.

Chapter 6, "Mastering Keto Cooking Techniques" introduces you to a variety of cooking techniques that make preparing keto meals a breeze.

Chapter 7, "Delicious, Easy-to-Follow Keto Recipes," provides a compilation of satisfying, easy-to-make recipes, designed to keep you in a state of ketosis without compromising on taste.

Chapter 8, "Overcoming Common Keto Challenges," addresses potential hurdles that you may face during your transition into the ketogenic lifestyle, and provides practical solutions to keep you on track.

In Chapter 9, "Keto and Exercise: A Comprehensive Guide," we explore how to integrate physical activities into your new lifestyle.

Chapter 10, "Keto for the Long Haul: Sustainability and Adaptation," provides guidance on maintaining your ketogenic lifestyle in the long term, offering tips on adapting it to various life situations.

Finally, Chapter 11, "Your Keto Lifestyle: Tips and Tricks for Success," equips you with additional tips, tricks, and advice to ensure you get the most out of your ketogenic journey.

Whether you are new to the concept of a ketogenic diet, or someone looking to deepen your understanding, this book aims to provide an easy-to-follow guide through every step of the process. From understanding the basics of keto, to maintaining it as a lifestyle, we got you covered. So, let's embark on this fascinating journey to wellness and vitality together!

Chapter 1
Understanding the Ketogenic Diet

In the world of nutrition and health, trends come and go. However, there are some that capture the world's attention and stand the test of time due to their profound effects on health and wellbeing. The ketogenic diet, popularly known as "keto," is one such trend that has proven to be more than just a passing fad. Before we dive into the nitty-gritty of the ketogenic lifestyle, it is crucial to lay a solid foundation of understanding. This chapter aims to provide that base, by unraveling the fundamental aspects of the ketogenic diet, its history, the process of ketosis, and the myriad of potential benefits it brings to the table.

1. Introduction to the Ketogenic Diet

At its core, the ketogenic diet is a low-carb, high-fat dietary plan. It aims to reprogram your body to use a different type of fuel. Instead of relying on sugar (glucose) that comes from carbohydrates (such as grains, legumes, vegetables, and fruits), the keto diet relies on ketone bodies, a type of fuel that the liver produces from stored fat.

In a typical Western diet, you're eating a lot of carbohydrates, and your body uses these for energy. However, if you limit the number of carbs you eat, your body has to find another source of energy, in this case, fat. This switch from a "carb-burning" state to a "fat-burning" state is what distinguishes the ketogenic diet from many other dieting methods and is what leads to many of its associated benefits.

But, the ketogenic diet isn't just about losing weight. Over the decades, a growing body of research suggests that it might help with a lot of other health issues too, including diabetes, heart disease, certain cancers, Alzheimer's disease, and more. It's important to note that many of these benefits are still under scientific review, and results may vary from person to person.

2. The History of the Ketogenic Diet

The roots of the ketogenic diet can be traced back to Ancient Greece, where physicians used fasting as a method to treat various illnesses. However, the diet as we know it today was developed in the 1920s as a treatment for epilepsy. At the time, researchers found that fasting improved the symptoms of epileptic patients, but fasting couldn't be maintained indefinitely. So, they developed the ketogenic diet to mimic the biochemical effects of fasting while allowing food intake. The diet fell out of favor for a while with the development of antiepileptic drugs but has seen a resurgence in recent years, due to its potential benefits for various health conditions.

3. Ketosis and Your Body

When you drastically reduce your carbohydrate intake, your body enters a metabolic state known as ketosis. In this state, the body has to burn fat for energy instead of glucose. This is because your body doesn't have enough carbohydrates to burn for energy. The liver converts this fat into ketones, a type of acid, which can be used by the body for fuel. It's important to note that achieving ketosis requires careful planning—eating too many carbs or too much protein can knock you out of ketosis.

4. The Benefits of the Ketogenic Diet

While the primary reason many people start the ketogenic diet is for weight loss, it has been observed to have several other potential health benefits. For example, it might help reduce the risk of developing certain diseases like diabetes and heart disease. It's also been studied for its potential effects on acne, brain diseases, and even cancer. Additionally, the diet may have benefits on mental health and physical performance.

Remember, while the ketogenic diet has potential benefits, it's not suitable for everyone, and you should consult a healthcare professional before starting.

5. Types of Ketogenic Diets

There are several versions of the ketogenic diet, each with varying levels of strictness:

The Standard Ketogenic Diet (SKD) is the most common and researched version. It typically contains 70-75% fat, 20% protein, and only 5-10% carbohydrates.

The Cyclical Ketogenic Diet (CKD) involves periods of higher-carb intake, such as 5 ketogenic days, followed by 2 high-carb days.

The Targeted Ketogenic Diet (TKD) allows you to add carbohydrates around workouts.

The High-Protein Ketogenic Diet is similar to the standard ketogenic diet, but with more protein. The ratio might be around 60% fat, 35% protein, and 5% carbs.

Each of these diets suits different people, depending on their health goals, activity levels, and lifestyle.

6. Foods to Eat and Avoid

It's essential to know what foods are permitted, and which ones to avoid, on a ketogenic diet. This is not a diet where you can 'wing it'. Planning and knowledge are key.

You will base most of your meals around these foods:

Meats: Red meat, steak, ham, sausage, bacon, chicken, and turkey
Fatty fish: Salmon, trout, tuna, and mackerel
Eggs: Pastured or omega-3 whole eggs
Butter and cream: Grass-fed when possible
Cheese: Unprocessed cheese
Nuts and seeds: Almonds, walnuts, flax seeds, pumpkin seeds, chia seeds, etc.
Healthy oils: Primarily extra virgin olive oil, coconut oil, and avocado oil
Avocados: Whole avocados or freshly made guacamole
Low-carb veggies: Green veggies, tomatoes, onions, peppers, etc.

Foods you should avoid:

Sugary foods: Soda, fruit juice, smoothies, cake, ice cream, candy, etc.
Grains or starches: Wheat-based products, rice, pasta, cereal, etc.
Fruit: All fruit, except small portions of berries
Beans or legumes: Peas, kidney beans, lentils, chickpeas, etc.
Root vegetables and tubers: Potatoes, sweet potatoes, carrots, parsnips, etc.
Low-fat or diet products: These types of foods are often high in carbs.
Unhealthy fats: Limit your intake of processed vegetable oils, mayonnaise, etc.

7. Transitioning to the Ketogenic Diet

Switching to the ketogenic diet isn't always a smooth process. It can sometimes lead to side effects, collectively known as, the 'keto flu. Symptoms can include poor energy and mental function, increased hunger, sleep issues, nausea, and digestive discomfort. These symptoms are temporary, and there are ways to minimize or cure them, which we will discuss later in this book.

Even though the ketogenic diet is safe for healthy people, there may be some initial side effects while your body adapts. You need to remember that some people should not follow it without medical supervision.

8. Health Considerations and Precautions

While the ketogenic diet can bring a multitude of potential health benefits, it's not suitable for everyone. Certain people should exercise caution and speak to their doctor before starting a ketogenic diet, including people with type 1 diabetes, pancreatic disease, liver conditions, thyroid problems, gallbladder disease or removal, a history of eating disorders, and pregnant or breastfeeding women.

Moreover, medications for diabetes and high blood pressure may need to be adjusted when you're on a ketogenic diet. If you take medication for any chronic health condition, speak to your doctor before starting the diet.

9. The Role of Hydration and Electrolytes

A crucial yet often overlooked aspect of the ketogenic diet is hydration and electrolyte balance. Since a ketogenic diet acts as a natural diuretic, it's easy to lose water and electrolytes quickly. Staying well-hydrated and maintaining electrolyte balance is key in reducing potential side effects like keto flu, cramps, and constipation. Drinking plenty of water, consuming foods high in sodium, potassium, and magnesium, or considering an electrolyte supplement, can help.

10. Monitoring Ketosis

There are several ways to know if you're in ketosis. These include weight loss, increased ketones in the blood, breath, or urine, reduced appetite, increased focus and energy, short-term fatigue, short-term decrease in performance, digestive issues, and insomnia. You can also use a device like a glucometer to measure your blood ketone levels precisely.

11. Keto and Sustainability

Some critics argue that diets like the keto diet are hard to stick to due to their restrictive nature. While it's true that sticking to a low-carb, high-fat diet can be challenging for some, it's definitely not impossible. Strategies such as meal planning, mindful eating, finding low-carb substitutes for your favorite high-carb foods, and getting support from friends or online communities, can all make sticking to a keto diet more manageable.

12. Keto Adaptation: The Transition Phase

When you first start a ketogenic diet, your body has to go through a transition phase to switch from burning glucose to burning fat for energy, known as keto adaptation. This process can take anywhere from a few days to a few weeks, depending on your body's metabolism. During this time, you may experience what is commonly known as the "keto flu," a group of symptoms, including fatigue, nausea, headaches, and irritability. However, these symptoms are temporary and are a sign that your body is adapting to burning fat for fuel.

13. Ketogenic Diet and Exercise

One common misconception about the ketogenic diet is that it hampers exercise performance due to the reduction of carbohydrate intake. However, that's not entirely accurate. While some athletes may experience a temporary decrease in performance during the initial keto adaptation phase, most can maintain their usual routine. Moreover, for endurance exercises, a ketogenic diet can be beneficial as the body utilizes fat, an abundant energy source. It's essential, however, to listen to your body and adjust your activity levels as needed.

14. Common Mistakes When Starting a Ketogenic Diet

Starting a new diet, especially one that involves a drastic change in your eating habits like the ketogenic diet, can be challenging. Common mistakes include not eating enough fat, consuming too much protein, not considering micronutrients, not drinking enough water or neglecting electrolyte balance, and not giving your body time to adapt before making changes. It's important to remember, like any lifestyle change, the ketogenic diet requires a learning curve.

15. The Role of Intermittent Fasting in the Ketogenic Diet

Intermittent fasting involves cycling between periods of eating and fasting, and can be an effective strategy in conjunction with a ketogenic diet. Fasting helps facilitate ketosis as your body depletes its glucose reserves and starts burning fat for energy. However, it's important to approach intermittent fasting with caution and knowledge, as doing it incorrectly can lead to adverse health effects.

16. Understanding Net Carbs

In a ketogenic diet, keeping a check on your carbohydrate intake is essential. But it's not just any type of carbohydrates - it's net carbs that matter. Net carbs are the total carbohydrates in foods, minus the fiber content. Fiber is a type of carbohydrate that our bodies can't digest, so it doesn't raise blood sugar levels or interfere with ketosis. Therefore, when counting carbs on a ketogenic diet, you only need to consider net carbs. Many foods, like vegetables, may seem high in carbs, but much of it is fiber, so their impact on your blood sugar and ketosis is minimal.

17. The Role of Fat Quality in a Ketogenic Diet

The quality of fat in your diet matters. Opting for healthy fats is essential on a ketogenic diet. Monounsaturated and saturated fats should form the bulk of your fat intake. These can come from sources like avocados, olive oil, nuts, seeds, and high-fat dairy. Trans fats and processed polyunsaturated fats, usually found in processed foods and fried items, should be avoided.

18. Potential Long-term Effects of a Ketogenic Diet

Research into the long-term effects of a ketogenic diet is ongoing. It's currently understood that while a ketogenic diet can lead to significant weight loss and improvements in blood sugar control, blood pressure, and cholesterol levels in the short term, long-term adherence may have potential risks, such as nutrient deficiencies, liver problems, and mood changes. Therefore, periodic assessments with a healthcare professional is recommended.

19. Customizing the Ketogenic Diet to Your Lifestyle

No diet is one-size-fits-all, and the ketogenic diet is no different. It's essential to tailor your ketogenic diet to fit your lifestyle, preferences, and health goals. This might mean choosing a less strict version of the diet, using supplements, or incorporating more variety into your meals. The goal is to make the diet sustainable for you in the long run.

20. Importance of a Support System

Having a support system can make a big difference when it comes to diet success. Surrounding yourself with supportive people who understand and respect your dietary choices can make your keto journey easier. Online communities, like keto forums and social media groups, can also be great places to find support, ask questions, and share your experiences.

Understanding the ketogenic diet is an essential first step on your journey towards better health. In the following chapters, we'll delve deeper into the practical aspects of starting, maintaining, and optimizing the ketogenic diet for your specific needs and circumstances.

Keto Made Simple

When following a ketogenic diet, calculating and fine-tuning your optimal macronutrient ratios, can help ensure you stay in ketosis and meet your health goals. While general keto macros are around 70-80% fat, 15-20% protein, and 5-10% carbs, your personal needs may vary. Factors like your activity levels, body composition goals, health conditions, and metabolic factors, can all impact your macros. Many experts suggest starting with standard keto ratios and making adjustments as needed, over time, based on your response. Apps, online calculators, and tracking can help dial in your optimal macros.

Low-carb doesn't mean leaving out all veggies! In fact, adding plenty of above-ground, leafy greens and certain other vegetables, can ensure a nutritious keto diet. Some excellent keto veggie choices include spinach, kale, lettuce, cucumbers, broccoli, cauliflower, zucchini, cabbage, asparagus, mushrooms, and more. Starchy root veggies like potatoes,carrots, corn, peas, and beans are best avoided. Getting creative with veggie-based meals, can make keto sustainable long-term.

Cravings for sweets, carbs, and comfort foods are common, especially when first starting keto. There are strategies to help manage these urges: drink water and get electrolytes when a craving strikes, eat enough fat and protein to stay satiated, distract yourself with activity, or wait 20 minutes until a craving passes. Good replacements for these high-carb foods are keto-approved snacks, like nuts, cheese, or avocados. Schedule higher-carb days if you're doing cyclical keto, and use keto substitutes for carbs like zoodles and cauliflower rice. To help avoid temptation, don't keep high-carb foods at home, manage stress, and get quality sleep. Cravings usually subside once keto adaptation occurs. Be prepared with keto snacks, and stay motivated!

Eating keto doesn't mean you have to avoid restaurants entirely. With some savvy menu choices, you can dine out, and stick to your plan. Some tasty options are grilled, baked, or broiled proteins like fish, chicken, or steak, extra veggies instead of starchy sides like rice or potatoes, salads with olive oil dressing sand added protein ; zoodles or mushroom noodles to replace pasta; and fresh berries with whipped cream for dessert.Be mindful of hidden carbs in sauces, dressings, and batter. Planning ahead when possible, and asking questions about preparation, can make eating out while doing keto very possible.

Feeling tired, sluggish, or foggy-headed is common during the initial adaptation phase, as your body gets used to using fat and ketones for energy. Here are some ways to help combat it: ensure adequate electrolytes and hydration; optimize protein intake - too little protein causes fatigue; add MCT oil or exogenous ketones; make sure you're not excessively restricting calories; manage stress and get quality sleep; get moving with light exercise to energize. Give it time - it usually resolves within 4–6 weeks once adapted. See your doctor if fatigue persists to check for underlying conditions.

Sustaining ketosis long-term requires consistency and lifestyle adaptation. Here are tips: Make gradual, maintainable changes to your diet and lifestyle; prepare weekly keto meal plans ahead of time; make sure you're eating enough with sufficient calories and nutrients; find substitutes for your favorite high-carb treats; incorporate new keto recipes frequently to prevent boredom; schedule "keto breaks" if following very low-carb keto; develop a routine and environment optimized for keto adherence; get support from friends, family, or online keto communities; stay focused on your motivation and the overall benefits. It takes dedication, but keto can become second nature over time.

Becoming "fat adapted" means training your body to burn fat more efficiently for fuel. This is a key goal on a keto diet. Here's how it works. Keeping carbs low and protein moderate, keeps insulin levels low. Low insulin triggers the release of fat from cells and signals the liver to produce ketones. As ketones rise, they become the primary fuel source, reducing blood sugar dependence. Cells and tissues adapt to using ketones and fatty acids, instead of glucose. The body becomes adept at mobilizing and burning stored body fat and dietary fat. Also,metabolic flexibility, when your body switches between the ability to burn carbs, fat and ketones, improves. The more adapted you are, the easier sticking to keto becomes.

The gut microbiome plays an important role in health and can be affected by diet. Here's how keto may impact gut bacteria. Very low-carb diets can reduce microbial diversity due to lack of dietary fiber. Keto diets favor certain bacteria, like Akkermansia, that thrive on fat, and ketones may provide an alternative energy source for microbes. Prebiotics from low-carb veggies feed beneficial bacteria, and probiotic foods can replenish good bacteria like kimchi, kefir, or yogurt. Resistant starches help feed microbes. Balancing prebiotic fiber, probiotics, and carb cycling, may help optimize your microbiome on keto.

Keto can cause short-term increases in LDL and total cholesterol, but its effect on heart health is complex: LDL rises due to increased transport of fat - large, fluffy LDL is benign; HDL (good) cholesterol rises, improving cholesterol ratio. Triglycerides decrease significantly, arterial plaque and inflammation may decrease, and blood pressure and blood sugar improve, thus reducing cardiac risk factors. Changes beyond total LDL cholesterol must be considered for heart disease risk. Always consult your doctor.

Many foods secretly contain more carbs than they appear. Watch out for: Sweeteners like sugar alcohols, maple syrup, honey; dairy such as, milk, yogurt, flavored creamers, and sauces and condiments, like barbecue, teriyaki, ketchup, and dressings. Drinks, such as flavored sodas, juices, smoothies, and alcohol mixes, can sneak in carbs as well. Snack foods, like crackers, pretzels, granola bars, and chips, are also notorious for hiding carbs. Fast foods, including nuggets, fried shells, and biscuits are known for slipping in extra carbs, and even nutritional bars can be full of unwanted carbohydrates. Seasonings, such as sweet BBQ rubs, marinades, and taco seasoning, may taste delicious, but not only are they full of so many unneeded extras, they are also filled with sodium.Scrutinize labels, measure portions, and track intake to account for hidden carbs.

Combining keto with resistance training, like weightlifting, can augment muscle development and fat lossMuscle burns more calories than fat, and it boosts metabolism. Lifting weights maintains muscle mass when losing weight, and resistance training triggers the release of fat-burning hormones. Ketones may provide an alternative muscle fuel source, while post-workout protein supports muscle growth and recovery. Aim for 2-4 lifting sessions per week, along with ketogenic nutrition.

Tracking key numbers provides insight into your nutritional ketosis and how your body is responding.Monitor your daily fat, protein, and net carbs. Make sure you're not at too great a deficit with calories,Remember, blood meter readings will indicate your level of ketosis. pre- and post-meal blood sugar numbers, and provides carb tolerance.You can gauge fat loss and muscle gain with weight, and changes in inches reflect body recomposition. Keep in mind, you need to have your cholesterol levels checked occasionally. All of this tracking can help fine-tune your keto plan, for optimal results.

While technically keto-friendly, certain ultra-processed foods may negatively impact health. Prioritize: Organic, pasture-raised animal foods whenever possible; wild caught, low-mercury fish and seafood; organic dairy and eggs from free-range sources; fresh or frozen vegetables over canned varieties; avocado, olive, coconut, and nut oils over seed oils; nut and seed butters without added oils; 90% or higher dark chocolate for lower sugar; nuts, seeds and berries over refined snacks. Keto requires fat - be mindful of its source.

Drinking on keto is possible but requires caution: Count carb and calories in beer, wine, spirits, and mixers; dry wines or straight liquors are the lowest carb options;avoid sweet mixers. Limiting alcohol consumption is truly the best choice because it pauses ketosis until the liver processes it.However, if you do choose to have a drink, try to hydrate before and after because alcohol is very dehydrating.Be prepared for lower alcohol tolerance, especially if you're new to keto.With mindfulness, an occasional drink can fit into a keto lifestyle.

Traveling while on keto may seem daunting, but you can keep up your keto on vacation. Research restaurant menus in the area ahead of time,pack snacks and portable keto foods if you'll be on the go, and request a mini-fridge in your hotel for basics like cheese and nuts. When booking flights, request a low-carb meal option,scope out nearby grocery stores to stock up on staples, and bring electrolyte supplements.Traveling can be dehydrating, but with prep and planning, you don't have to put your diet on hold for travel.

Helping friends and family understand the keto diet can enable your success. Explain the mechanisms and how ketosis and fat burning work. Share research and resources supporting keto's benefits,offer to cook a keto-friendly meal to demonstrate, or suggest trying keto for a short trial. Emphasize that it's your own, educated choice, and ask them to respect your dietary needs. Encourage questions because open communication is key! With education and support, they're likely to come around.

Working shifts can complicate meal timing and sleep. Here are some tips for keto success. Pack snacks like nuts and cheese to fuel erratic shifts, and make sure to meal prep on days off, for quick grab-and-go eats.Opt for simple, repeatable meals to reduce decision fatigue, and focus on good sleep habits between work days. Always prioritize rest. Consider cyclical keto to allow meals right after night shifts , and don't forget to manage stress. With planning, keto can work with an irregular schedule.

The metabolic changes of menopause can make weight and hunger management more difficult. Here's how keto can help: Stabilizing blood sugar reduces insulin spikes and cravings; appetite regulation promotes intuitive eating; utilizing body fat for fuel stabilizes energy, despite hormone shifts; low-carb and healthy fats support heart health; ketones provide an alternative brain fuel to combat fogginess; and reduced inflammation helps manage joint pain and hot flashes. Keto's effects on hormones, hunger, and metabolism can support women through menopause.

Some argue that keto harms the planet due to high meat and dairy intake. Ways to increase sustainability: Source quality animal foods locally or from regenerative farms when possible; limit intake of beef and lamb which have the highest climate impact; incorporate organ meats - using the whole animal reduces waste; eat more plant-based keto meals focused on nuts, seeds and avocados; reduce food waste by meal planning and using leftovers; and choose seafood options with responsible, ethical harvesting practices. With awareness, keto can be modified to be friendlier for the environment.

Intuitive eating means listening to internal hunger cues instead of external food rules. Here's how to make keto more intuitive: Eat when hungry, - pause when full; allow satiating high fat foods instead of avoiding fat or calories; add carbohydrates if your body is signaling a need for them; don't label foods inherently "good" or "bad" - focus on how they make your body feel; focus on nutrition and health, not conforming to keto dogma; and give yourself unconditional permission to eat food that fuels you. Tuning in to your body's signals is key for sustainable keto success.

Some medications may require dose adjustments or additional monitoring on keto: Diabetes medications - lowered blood sugar may increase risk of hypoglycemia; hypertension meds - lower blood pressure often allows dose reduction; statins - increased LDL may require cholesterol monitoring and dosage changes; anticonvulsants - ketosis may alter medication levels, so monitoring is advised; lithium - dehydration and electrolyte shifts may impact therapy; thyroid hormones - thyroid panels should be evaluated periodically. Always discuss keto with your doctor, especially if you're taking medications.

A healthy gut microbiome is linked to overall wellbeing. To nourish your gut on keto: Eat plenty of non-starchy vegetables which provide prebiotic fiber, and consider resistant starches via carb cycling to feed gut flora. Incorporate probiotic foods like kimchi, kefir, and sauerkraut, and stay well hydrated to manage constipation if it arises. Limit use of antibiotics, NSAIDs, and processed foods when possible.Manage stress levels through lifestyle because stress definitely impacts gut balance. Supporting gut bacteria diversity may benefit mental and metabolic health.

A metallic, fruity odor on the breath is common in ketosis. Causes include: Acetone buildup - ketones expelled through breathing; dehydration - lack of water reduces saliva production; gut flora imbalance - bacteria produce odorous compounds; post-meal protein breakdown. Solutions include: Stay hydrated and drink water with meals; use breath mints, gum or mouthwash, after eating; try digestive enzymes to ease protein breakdown; consume chlorophyll-rich foods, like spinach, to mask odors; wait it out - keto breath usually resolves in a few weeks as the body adapts. Keto breath may be unpleasant, but is a harmless side effect.

Body recomposition means losing fat and gaining muscle simultaneously. Keto tactics for recomposition include: Eating sufficient protein - aim for 0.6-1 gram per pound of lean mass; incorporating resistance training - lift weights 2–4 times per week; prioritizing sleep - poor sleep impacts muscle growth and fat loss; managing stress levels - cortisol inhibits recomposition; being patient and consistent - noticeable changes may take months; consider cyclical keto to support workout performance; track progress with measurements - weight may not change as muscle and fat shift. With strategic nutrition and training, keto can transform your physique.

The "keto flu" refers to temporary symptoms that may arise when transitioning into ketosis. Here's how to manage: Get plenty of rest - your body is undergoing major metabolic shifts; stay hydrated and replenish electrolytes, especially sodium; eat enough calories and nutrients - don't crash diet when starting keto; consider exogenous ketones or MCT oil, to give energy levels a boost; adjust activity levels if needed - intense workouts may need to wait; know it will pass - symptoms usually resolve within 1–2 weeks. Be patient through the adaptation phase to feel your best on keto long-term.

When starting keto, anticipate some trial and error: Response varies between individuals.What works for others may not be right for you. It can take weeks or longer for your body to become keto adapted., especially weight loss, are often not linear or steady, and suboptimal sleep, stress, or hormones can stall progress.The ideal carbohydrate threshold differs based on the individual, and keep in mind that occasional plateaus are normal - trust the process. Patience and self-compassion are key.

A common misconception is that low-carb eating must be expensive. Ways to save: Prioritize inexpensive proteins like eggs, whole chickens, fatty ground beef; buy frozen vegetables - they last longer than fresh; purchase fattier cuts of meat rather than lean; buy nuts, nut butters, and seeds in bulk; use coupons and shop sales for pricier items like cheese; stick to simple, repeatable meals rather than elaborate recipes. With planning, keto can fit any budget.

25

Chapter 2
The Science Behind Keto

The ketogenic diet has been under the limelight for the past few years, with people all around the world adopting this lifestyle for its profound benefits on weight loss, energy levels, and overall health. But what gives the ketogenic diet its power? What processes occur inside our bodies when we follow this diet? This chapter will unravel the science behind the ketogenic diet.

1. Understanding Metabolism: Glucose Versus Ketones

Metabolism, the process your body uses to convert food into energy, is central to understanding the science behind the ketogenic diet. The human body primarily relies on glucose, a type of sugar, for energy under normal dietary circumstances. We get glucose from carbohydrates found in foods like bread, pasta, fruits, and sugar. After eating, carbohydrates are broken down into glucose, which is then transported to cells throughout the body, to be used as energy.

But what happens when the availability of glucose is limited, as in the case of the ketogenic diet? This is where ketones come into play. When carbohydrate intake is drastically reduced, your body enters a metabolic state called ketosis, where it starts burning fat for energy instead of glucose. The liver turns this fat into ketones, a type of acid, which can be used by your body (including your brain) as an energy source.

2. What is Ketosis?

Ketosis is a natural metabolic state wherein the body uses fat as its primary fuel source instead of glucose. Under normal circumstances, our bodies are sugar-burning machines. However, when we limit our carbohydrate intake, our bodies are forced to find an alternate fuel source: fat. The process of breaking down fat for energy produces ketones, hence the name 'ketosis.'

Ketosis should not be confused with ketoacidosis, a dangerous condition often associated with type 1 diabetes. While both lead to increased production of ketones, ketoacidosis happens when the levels become too high, making the blood extremely acidic.

3. How does the Body Enter Ketosis?

Transitioning from a glucose-based metabolism to a ketone-based metabolism doesn't happen overnight. It requires a significant reduction in carbohydrate intake, usually less than 50 grams per day, alongside a high intake of fats. Once carbohydrate stores (glycogen) in the body are depleted, and the body recognizes that it needs another source of energy, it begins to break down fat, leading to the production of ketones for energy. This shift can take anywhere from a couple of days to a week or more, depending on the individual.

4. The Different Types of Ketones

When your body enters ketosis, it produces three types of ketones: Acetoacetate (AcAc), Beta-hydroxybutyric acid (BHB), and Acetone. AcAc is the first ketone produced during ketosis, some of which is then converted into BHB, the most abundant and energy-efficient ketone. Acetone is the least abundant, created as a byproduct of AcAc.

5. The Role of Insulin in Ketosis

Insulin is a hormone that plays a crucial role in metabolism. It allows cells in the body to take in glucose and use it as a source of energy, or store it for future use. When you eat a meal rich in carbohydrates, your blood glucose levels rise, leading to an increase in insulin release. Insulin acts to lower blood glucose levels by facilitating its uptake into cells.

In a ketogenic diet, because carbohydrate intake is drastically reduced, insulin levels drop, and fat stores are released into the bloodstream to be used as energy. Lower insulin levels also allow for the production of ketones, thus inducing a state of ketosis.

6. Benefits of Ketones

Ketones are a super fuel for our bodies. They provide numerous benefits that make them superior to glucose in many aspects. Ketones are an energy-efficient fuel source. They provide more energy per unit of oxygen used compared to glucose, leading to increased endurance and energy levels.

Moreover, ketones, particularly Beta-Hydroxybutyrate (BHB), have shown neuroprotective and anti-inflammatory effects. This could have potential benefits in managing conditions such as Alzheimer's, Parkinson's, and other neurological disorders.

7. The Brain on Ketones

The brain is a major organ that benefits from ketosis. Despite its small size relative to the rest of the body, the brain consumes a huge amount of energy daily. While the brain typically uses glucose as its primary fuel source, it can readily use ketones when glucose availability is limited.

In fact, during periods of fasting or strict carbohydrate restriction, up to 70% of the brain's energy can come from ketones. This ability to utilize ketones helps preserve brain function and protect against neural damage during periods of energy shortage.

8. The Impact of the Ketogenic Diet on Body Composition

The ketogenic diet has profound effects on body composition, mainly through its role in weight loss. By switching the body's metabolism from burning glucose to burning fat, the ketogenic diet helps people lose weight more efficiently compared to other diets. This is due to several reasons - the satiety effect of protein, the appetite-suppressing effect of ketones, and the drop in insulin levels that facilitate fat burning.

9. Keto and the Thermic Effect of Food

The Thermic Effect of Food (TEF), also known as diet-induced thermogenesis, refers to the energy expended by our bodies in processing food for use and storage. It varies depending on the macronutrient composition of our diets. Protein has a higher TEF compared to carbohydrates and fat, meaning your body burns more calories processing protein than the other macronutrients.

On a ketogenic diet, even though fat is the most consumed macronutrient, moderate protein consumption is also encouraged. This moderate protein intake, coupled with the low carbohydrate intake, can increase the thermic effect of food and enhance weight loss.

10. Understanding the Role of Leptin and Ghrelin

Leptin and Ghrelin are two hormones that play significant roles in energy balance and appetite regulation. Leptin, often referred to as the 'satiety hormone', is produced by fat cells and signals the brain to reduce appetite when we have sufficient fat stores. Ghrelin, on the other hand, is known as the 'hunger hormone'. It increases appetite and drives fat storage.

A well-formulated ketogenic diet can help regulate these hormones. Lower insulin levels from a reduced carbohydrate intake can improve leptin signaling. Additionally, the high fat and protein content of the ketogenic diet can keep ghrelin levels in check, thereby reducing feelings of hunger.

11. Keto and Gut Health

Emerging research suggests that a ketogenic diet can influence the gut microbiota, the community of microorganisms living in our intestines. A diverse and balanced gut microbiota is critical for overall health. Some studies have found that a ketogenic diet can increase the abundance of beneficial gut bacteria that are associated with weight loss and improved gut health.

12. The Impact of Keto on Cholesterol Levels

It's common to see an initial increase in cholesterol levels when starting a ketogenic diet. This is because as your body burns its stored fat, cholesterol is released into the bloodstream. However, long-term, well-formulated, ketogenic diets have been associated with improved cholesterol profiles, including lower LDL (bad) cholesterol and triglyceride levels and increased HDL (good) cholesterol levels.

13. The Science Behind Keto and Diabetes

For those with type 2 diabetes, the ketogenic diet can be a useful tool. By cutting out carbohydrates, blood sugar levels can be more easily controlled. Additionally, because the diet eliminates the sugar highs and crashes associated with a high-carb diet, it can help to reduce cravings and overeating.

The ketogenic diet can also have positive effects on insulin sensitivity. Many people with type 2 diabetes suffer from insulin resistance, a condition where the body isn't able to use insulin effectively to regulate blood sugar levels. The ketogenic diet can help to lower insulin levels and improve insulin sensitivity, leading to better blood sugar control.

14. Ketosis and Autophagy

Autophagy, from the Greek meaning 'self-eating', is a process where the body cleans out damaged cells and generates new, healthy ones. It's a crucial system used by your body to detoxify and recycle components, and it has links to longevity and disease prevention.

Ketosis can induce autophagy, which is typically triggered by nutrient deprivation. A well-formulated, ketogenic diet puts the body in a state similar to fasting, hence inducing this cellular cleanup process. This could potentially have benefits like improved brain function, immune system regulation, and aging delay.

15. The Science Behind Keto Flu

When first starting a ketogenic diet, some people may experience what's commonly referred to as the 'keto flu'. Symptoms can include headache, fatigue, nausea, dizziness, and irritability. This is your body's reaction to the drastic shift from a carbohydrate-based energy source to a fat-based one.

As your body depletes its glucose stores and begins to burn fat for fuel, it also begins to excrete more electrolytes than normal. This can lead to an electrolyte imbalance, causing the aforementioned symptoms. Rest, hydration, and replenishing electrolytes can alleviate these symptoms.

16. Keto and Hormone Regulation

A well-structured, ketogenic diet, can help with the regulation of hormones. For women, particularly those with Polycystic Ovary Syndrome (PCOS), keto can help regulate insulin, cortisol, and other hormone levels, improving symptoms.

Keto can also positively affect hormones like human growth hormone (HGH), a key player in growth, body composition, cell repair, and metabolism. Fasting and high-intensity exercise, both of which can be components of a keto lifestyle, can stimulate HGH production.

17. Keto and Cardiovascular Health

Research has shown potential benefits of a ketogenic diet on cardiovascular health. In addition to promoting weight loss and improving cholesterol levels, as mentioned earlier, keto has also been found to reduce high blood pressure in some individuals. High blood pressure is a significant risk factor for heart disease. By lowering blood pressure, the ketogenic diet could potentially reduce the risk of heart disease.

Moreover, by lowering insulin levels, a ketogenic diet can help reduce inflammation, another risk factor for heart disease. Chronic inflammation can damage the walls of the arteries, leading to plaque buildup and potentially causing heart disease.

18. Ketones and Endurance Performance

Keto-adaptation, the process where your body becomes efficient at burning fat and ketones, can be beneficial for endurance athletes. Once fully adapted, the body has access to a vast amount of stored fat for energy, compared to limited glycogen stores. This can prevent "bonking" or "hitting the wall," a common problem for endurance athletes relying on carbohydrates.

19. Nutrient Density on a Ketogenic Diet

While the ketogenic diet limits certain food groups, particularly grains and sugars, it doesn't mean that it's low in nutrients. In fact, a well-planned ketogenic diet can be quite nutrient-dense. Foods commonly included in a ketogenic diet, like leafy greens, avocados, nuts, seeds, and fatty fish, are rich in essential vitamins and minerals.

However, because of the restrictive nature of the diet, some people might need to take supplements to meet their micronutrient needs, especially for nutrients like calcium, magnesium, and certain B vitamins.

20. Neuroprotective Benefits of Ketones

The ketogenic diet was originally designed to treat epilepsy in the 1920s and is still used for this purpose today. This gives us an early indication of the diet's potential neuroprotective benefits. Research suggests that ketones provide a more efficient fuel source for the brain and can enhance mitochondrial function, leading to reduced oxidative stress and inflammation in the brain.

Apart from epilepsy, research into the effects of the ketogenic diet on other neurological disorders such as Alzheimer's disease, Parkinson's disease, and even brain cancer, is ongoing and showing promising results.

21. Future Directions in Ketogenic Research

The science behind the ketogenic diet is still evolving. Ongoing and future research, will continue to investigate its long-term safety and efficacy, potential applications in treating various diseases, mechanisms of action, and more. As our understanding of the diet and its effects on the body deepens, we can better utilize it as a tool for health and well-being.

22. Keto and Mental Health

Emerging research suggests that the ketogenic diet may offer benefits not just for the body, but also for the mind. Some studies have shown that the ketogenic diet may help reduce symptoms in people with mental health disorders, such as depression, bipolar disorder, and anxiety. The proposed mechanism is through reducing inflammation, improving mitochondrial function, and boosting BDNF (Brain-Derived Neurotrophic Factor), a protein that promotes brain health.

23. The Role of MCTs in Ketosis

Medium-chain triglycerides (MCTs) are a type of fat that's easily digested and absorbed by the body. MCTs are converted in the liver, into ketones, providing an immediate source of energy for the brain and muscles. This makes MCTs especially beneficial for those following a ketogenic diet, as they can help enhance ketone production and maintain a state of ketosis.

24. Keto Diet and Cancer Research

There's growing interest in the potential role of the ketogenic diet as an adjuvant therapy in cancer treatment. The premise is that cancer cells primarily use glucose for energy. By restricting carbohydrates and thereby reducing blood glucose levels, the ketogenic diet may "starve" the cancer cells and inhibit their growth.

While the research is still in the early stages and mostly limited to animal studies, the results are promising. However, it's important to note that the ketogenic diet should not replace conventional cancer treatments, but can be considered as part of a comprehensive treatment plan under the supervision of healthcare professionals.

25. Keto and Lifespan

Recent research has been exploring the potential link between a ketogenic diet and lifespan extension. Some animal studies have shown that a ketogenic diet can increase lifespan and improve healthspan, the period during which one is generally healthy and free from serious disease.

It's believed that the diet's ability to induce ketosis and autophagy, reduce inflammation, and improve metabolic health are reasons to consider this type of lifestyle., It modulates aging pathways, like the mTOR and AMPK, and this can contribute to all the other wonderful benefits of keto. However, more research, especially long-term human studies, are needed to fully understand these potential effects.

26. The Versatility of Keto Diet

The ketogenic diet is highly versatile and can be tailored to meet individual needs and preferences. Variations of the diet, such as the cyclic ketogenic diet (CKD), targeted ketogenic diet (TKD), and high-protein ketogenic diet, offer more flexibility, allowing individuals to incorporate more carbohydrates around workouts. Switching between variations would help to make the diet more sustainable in the long term.

This concludes our deep dive into the science behind the ketogenic diet. As you can see, the ketogenic diet is more than just a weight-loss tool. Its wide-ranging impacts on various aspects of health underline the transformative potential that dietary change can bring about. Remember, knowledge is the key to success. Understanding the science behind the diet can empower you to make informed decisions and fully harness the benefits of the diet for your health and well-being.

Along with all the appreciated views of the keto diet, there are a few criticisms. You will find these listed below

27. Criticism: Keto aggravates gout.

Concerns about keto worsening gout arise because ketosis raises uric acid levels temporarily. However, research shows that adhering to a keto diet for 3–6 months can lower uric acid back to normal range. Additionally, keto elimination of sugar and grain carbohydrates and emphasis on whole foods may reduce inflammation - a key factor in gout. Nonetheless, those with a history of gout should proceed cautiously with medical guidance when starting keto

28. Criticism: Keto causes headaches.

Headaches can occur temporarily when first transitioning to keto due to electrolyte/mineral imbalance, as ketones flush water and electrolytes from the body. Headache frequency resolves for most within 1–2 weeks. Supporting electrolyte status with extra sodium, magnesium, and potassium supplementation, can help minimize headaches and other "keto flu" symptoms. Staying well-hydrated is also crucial.

29.Criticism: The ketogenic diet is just a fad.

Arguments that keto is just another diet fad are simply untrue. The diet's origins date back to the 1920s, when it was developed to control seizures. The ketogenic diet is supported by decades of research and clinical applications demonstrating efficacy for a range of health conditions. While popularity has fluctuated, the diet was never fully abandoned due to continued acknowledgment of its benefits by physicians and patients.

30. Criticism: Keto causes bad breath.

This phenomenon, nicknamed "keto breath," can occur on very low-carb ketogenic diets, especially early on. Acetone, a ketone body produced in ketosis, is eliminated through breath and urine, causing a fruity odor in some. Staying hydrated and using breath mints or oral hygiene products can help. As the body adapts, acetone levels normalize and breath odor subsides.

The arguments against the ketogenic diet, while worth addressing, do not detract from the wealth of scientific evidence demonstrating safety and diverse benefits when the diet is properly implemented. Vigilance around individual factors like kidney function, thyroid status, cholesterol levels, and micronutrient intake, allows for safe, long-term adherence. Like any diet, considerations and precautions may apply to some individuals. However, the benefits seem to outweigh the potential risks for most people.

The Ketogenic Diet as a Cancer Therapy

The use of the ketogenic diet as an adjuvant cancer treatment is an emerging area of research that is showing promising results. Cancer cells thrive on glucose. The ketogenic diet is thought to literally "starve" tumor cells, as it restricts carbohydrates and lowers blood glucose levels. This antitumor effect has been demonstrated in animal models and some human studies. Additionally, ketones themselves may directly inhibit cancer progression and metastasis. However, more research is still needed on optimal implementation of keto as a cancer therapy.

Potential Use for Diabetes Prevention

With its potent effects on stabilizing blood sugar, sensitizing cells to insulin, lowering inflammation, and encouraging weight loss, the ketogenic diet may also play a future role in preventing or delaying the onset of type 2 diabetes. By targeting underlying insulin resistance early, keto could hypothetically stop the disease process before it escalates to full-blown diabetes. This potential application requires longer-term randomized controlled trials, but is logically based on the diet's anti-diabetic mechanisms.

Effects on NON-Alcoholic Fatty Liver Disease

Emerging data highlights the potential for ketogenic diets to improve or reverse fatty liver, a condition involving excess fat accumulation in liver cells. This steatosis can progress to dangerous inflammation and liver dysfunction. By lowering liver fat, ketosis may significantly reduce fatty liver disease. This is attributed to enhanced fat burning, reduced lipogenesis, decreased insulin resistance, and lowered inflammation from the diet.

The Gut Microbiome's Role in Ketogenic Diets

There is a complex interplay between the diet and the community of microorganisms residing in the gastrointestinal tract, known as the gut microbiota. Research indicates that the unique gut microbiome signature of an individual may influence their response to a ketogenic diet. Future keto protocols could be further personalized by analyzing how the gut microbiome is impacted. Targeted use of pro- and prebiotics may further enhance results.

Can Keto Help Reduce Anxiety?

Scientific studies are now also exploring how ketogenic diets may alleviate anxiety disorders. One study found reduced anxiety in rats, which were fed a ketogenic diet. The antianxiety effect was associated with increased parasympathetic tone and gamma-aminobutyric acid (GABA) signaling in the brain. The diet may reduce inflammation and promote brain energy metabolism, but human trials are needed to further investigate keto's anxiolytic effects.

Ketone Esters: The Future of Ketosis?

Exogenous ketone supplements, like ketone esters and salts, allow users to get into ketosis faster while still consuming some carbohydrates. With keto popularity surging, the market for exogenous ketones is rapidly growing. However, costs are still prohibitive. Advances in the coming years will hopefully allow for increased production and affordability of exogenous ketones, unlocking faster, more convenient ketogenic protocols.

Leveraging the Power of MCT Oil

MCT oil and other medium chain triglyceride supplements have become staples for keto dieters due to their unique properties. Unlike long-chain fats, MCTs don't require bile acids or carnitine transport to be digested. They are taken up directly by the liver and readily converted to ketones. MCT oil provides an immediate and reliable way to raise ketone levels without carbohydrate restriction.

Using Keto Cycling Strategies

"Cyclical" ketogenic diet protocols involve strategically reintroducing higher carb periods into a ketogenic framework. Circumventing physical performance declines from long-term keto adaptation.However, cyclical keto regimens allow athletes to harness the power of ketosis, while maintaining high intensity training output. The higher carb periods also promote muscle growth, when paired with strength training.

Keto for Bodybuilding & Performance

Bodybuilders and physique competitors are increasingly beginning the keto diet, to simultaneously drop body fat and maintain lean muscle mass. Shorter cyclical keto is especially popular for enhancing the coveted shredded look before competitions. The beta-hydroxybutyrate (BHB) form of ketones may support hypertrophy and mitigate catabolism. When properly executed, keto shows major promise for aesthetic goals.

Timing of Meals and Carbohydrates

Emerging research suggests meal timing on keto diets may impact outcomes. One study found front-loading carbs in the first half of the day led to better blood sugar stability and cholesterol values versus spreading carbs evenly throughout the day. Another study concluded, consuming carbs at dinner only, did not sustain ketosis as well as breakfast-only carbs. More research is needed to confirm optimal carb timing.

Potential Longevity Effects

Data from animal models consistently shows ketogenic diets extending lifespan and . healthspan. This longevity boost is thought to stem from keto's effects on metabolism, oxidative stress, inflammation, Insulin-like growth factor-1 (IGF-1), and pathways involved in aging. Dietary ketosis mimics certain aspects of calorie restriction. Though human data is lacking, the anti-aging effects seen in animal studies are promising.

Enhancing Mitochondrial Function

A crucial anti-aging effect of the ketogenic diet involves enhancing mitochondrial health and efficiency. The diet promotes mitochondrial biogenesis, helping cells produce new mitochondria. Ketones also increase electron transport chain activity and ATP synthesis in existing mitochondria. Better functioning mitochondria translate to improved energy production, with less oxidative damage.

The Role of mTOR Inhibition

The enzyme, mTOR, acts as a key regulator of metabolism, cell growth, proliferation, and survival. Chronic mTOR over activation has been linked to diseases of aging. Animal research suggests ketogenic diets inhibit mTOR, which may underlie lifespan extension, decreased cancer progression, and other benefits. This again mimics effects of calorie restriction on healthspan.

Optimizing the Keto Macronutrient Ratio

There is no single ideal macronutrient ratio for the ketogenic diet. However, very high protein with insufficient fat reduces ketosis. Meanwhile, excessive calories from fat can also impair results. A general guideline for macronutrients is 60-75% calories from fat, 15-30% from protein, and 5-10% from carbs. But, optimal ratios differ based on individual factors.

Genetic Factors Influencing Response

A growing area of research is examining how genetics influence physiological response to ketogenic diets. Several polymorphisms have been identified that may affect keto response. For example, a mutation impairing fat breakdown could hinder ketone production. Other gene variants may predispose some to keto flu symptoms or alter cholesterol response. Nutrigenetic testing may inform personalized protocols.

Potential Benefits for Alzheimer's Disease

Because of its distinct metabolic effects and ability to provide an alternative fuel for the brain, the ketogenic diet is being studied as a nutritional strategy to prevent and manage Alzheimer's disease. The diet may reduce amyloid-beta accumulation and protect neurons from oxidative damage. So far, animal research and limited human trials demonstrate promising effects on Alzheimer's biomarkers.

Cholesterol Particle Size Matters

Several factors, beyond just total cholesterol, provide a clearer picture of heart disease risk. On keto diets, LDL particle size often shifts from small, dense LDL to large, "fluffy" LDL, which is less atherogenic. HDL cholesterol also increases. Additionally, LDL particles contain protective antioxidants on keto. For these reasons, elevated total cholesterol, alone, should not prompt alarm.

Ketogenic Strategies for Weight Maintenance

Adhering to keto long-term after reaching goal weight can be challenging. However, there are strategies to make weight maintenance more feasible. Incorporating occasional higher carb days, targeting carbohydrates around workouts, embracing a modified Mediterranean keto diet, and intermittent fasting, are just some options that may help sustain progress.

Keto Made Simple

Pick Your Intermittent Fasting Protocol

Intermittent fasting synergistically complements a well-formulated ketogenic diet. Options like 16:8, alternate day fasting, 24-hour fasts, and multi-day fasts, can be incorporated as needed, to boost ketone levels, accelerate fat burning, and stimulate autophagy. The flexibility of intermittent fasting makes it easy to find a protocol sustainable for the individual.

Is Fruit Off Limits on Keto Diets?

Limited fruit can be incorporated into a ketogenic diet, but choices must be very low sugar. Berries offer fiber, antioxidants, and phytonutrients while containing only minimal carbohydrates and not disrupting ketosis. However, moderation is still key, and most fruits should be viewed as occasional treats. Low-carb swaps can satisfy fruit cravings.

Beware of Hidden Carb Sources

Achieving and sustaining ketosis requires diligence, as carbs can sneak in from unexpected places. Foods assumed to be safe, like nuts, dairy products, and low-carb tortillas and bars, can sometimes contain hidden sugars. Review labels carefully and be cautious with processed foods marketed as "keto." Stick to, naturally low-carb, whole foods, as much as possible.

Don't Overdo Protein Intake

Dietary protein contains around 50% carbohydrates, as amino acids. Excessive protein intake can interfere with ketosis, as the body converts the amino acids into glucose via gluconeogenesis. Additionally, overeating protein on keto can strain the kidneys. Active individuals are likely need more protein, but intake should still be modulated, with fat making up the majority of calories.

Add Movement and Exercise

A ketogenic diet paired with regular exercise provides even more profound benefits. The diet fuels activity by giving muscles an abundant and steady energy supply. Activity further enhances insulin sensitivity, mitochondrial function, metabolism, body composition, and cellular cleanup processes. Even light movement supports overall health on keto.

Managing Keto with Diabetes Medications

Diabetic medications, especially insulin, may require adjustments on a ketogenic diet due to lowered glucose levels. Work closely with the healthcare team to avoid hypoglycemia. Likely, insulin and sulfonylurea doses will need reducing. Other agents, like SGLT-2 inhibitors, may also need their dosage and timing reassessed for safety on a keto diet.

Is Keto Safe for Prediabetes?

In prediabetes, blood sugar rises higher than normal but not high enough for a diabetes diagnosis. For prediabetics, keto's ability to lower fasting glucose, HbA1c, insulin levels, and insulin resistance may help halt progression to overt type 2 diabetes. However, keto for prediabetes should be overseen by a medical provider, as the diet and medication effects require careful review.

Beware the High Protein Trap

Many make the mistake of following a very high protein, low-carb diet without sufficient fat. However, without adequate dietary fat, the body lacks the substrate to make ketones. High protein intake also stresses the liver and kidneys and raises insulin. For successful keto diets, calories should come predominantly from fat with sufficient protein for muscle maintenance.

Keto Compared to the Mediterranean Diet

The Mediterranean and ketogenic diets are two popular nutrition approaches with compelling evidence bases. Each provides distinct benefits. Research is now looking at modified keto and Med diets that integrate aspects of both. A keto Mediterranean approach, focusing on whole foods, plant fats like olive oil, and seafood, may yield advantages of each diet.

Uncovering the Ideal Fat Sources

While keto is high fat, fat quality matters for optimal health. Dietary fats fall along a spectrum from very safe to clearly problematic. Focusing on predominantly unsaturated, anti-inflammatory fats, like olive oil, avocado, nuts, seeds, and fatty fish, is best. Minimizing processed, isolated fats is also wise. Variety across fat sources is key.

The Importance of Meal Planning for Success

Careful meal planning is crucial for long-term keto adherence. Planning out daily menus, batch cooking staples, like hard-boiled eggs and roasted veggies, and having snacks on hand, prevents cheating and burnout. Apps, websites, cookbooks, and other resources provide meal ideas and nutrition info. Make planning and prep part of your weekly routine.

Is Alcohol Compatible with Ketosis?

Limited alcohol can be worked into a keto lifestyle, but moderation and smart choices are critical. Dry wines, champagne, and clear liquors have low residual carbs and won't drastically impact ketosis. Beer and sweet mixers should be avoided. Overall alcohol intake should be minimized, as alcohol pauses fat burning, stresses the liver, and provides empty calories.

Managing Keto with Metabolic Conditions

For those with conditions like obesity, metabolic syndrome, insulin resistance, hypertension, and hyperlipidemia, keto can provide dramatic benefits by addressing root causes. However, close medical supervision is required when combining keto with medications for these conditions, as dosages will likely need adjusting to prevent side effects.

What About Calories on Keto?

Total caloric intake still matters on ketogenic diets. Although monitoring carbs, protein, and fat intake is priority, excessive calories from any source can hinder fat loss. Use a moderate caloric deficit of 15-30% below maintenance levels for steady, sustainable weight reduction. Track intake diligently, especially with calorically dense nuts, oils, and dairy.

Should You Try Exogenous Ketones?

Supplements providing direct exogenous sources of ketones, like ketone salts and esters, can rapidly elevate blood ketones even without dietary carbohydrate restriction. They may help mitigate keto flu symptoms, enhance cognition, boost athletic performance, and accelerate fat burning. However, costs are currently very high, and most people succeed without exogenous ketones.

Managing Cravings and Hunger on Keto

Cravings and hunger are common complaints initially when transitioning to keto, as the body is accustomed to running on carbs. However, once keto-adapted, cravings usually subside due to stabilization of blood sugar and insulin. Protein and fat provide satiety. If urges persist, examine triggers and diet composition. Increase fat calories if you're still hungry.

Is Keto Bad for the Gallbladder?

In rare cases, rapid weight loss from keto may cause temporary gallbladder distention, if bile production increases substantially. However, this risk is low on well-formulated, keto diets. Studies indicate keto improves gallbladder emptying compared to high-carb diets. Most importantly, consistently meeting fat intake needs, with a moderate caloric reduction, prevents gallbladder issues.

Leveraging Keto's Appetite Suppression

Keto Made Simple

One advantage of ketosis for weight loss, is reduced appetite, due to higher satiety from protein and fat, as well as appetite-regulating effects of ketones. Ghrelin and leptin, hormones that control hunger and satiety, are optimized on keto. Allow your natural hunger signals to guide food intake. It is not necessary or advisable to force-feed if you're not hungry while on keto.

Is Keto Good for Fertility and PCOS?

Insulin resistance and obesity underlie polycystic ovary syndrome (PCOS), a top cause of female infertility. By lowering insulin levels, decreasing inflammation, improving ovulation, and aiding weight loss, the ketogenic diet helps normalize hormonal dysfunction to improve fertility in PCOS. Keto also shows promise for enhancing outcomes in IVF.

Designing a Keto Diet for Diabetics

When formulating keto for diabetics, factors that impact blood sugar, like protein,fat type, and timing, deserve consideration. Some important strategies include limiting protein portions, choosing high MUFA fats, and properly spacing out meals. Individualizing carbohydrate amounts and timing is also key for glycemic control. Close medical management is imperative.

Is the Keto Flu Avoidable?

Because keto flu stems from electrolyte/mineral depletion, as ketones flush water from the body, preventing these transient symptoms is possible. Drinking bouillon or electrolyte beverages and supplementing with extra sodium, potassium, and magnesium, helps avert flu-like symptoms. Still, some discomfort adjusting to fat burning is unavoidable, but proper preparation minimizes misery.

Ketogenic Diets for Epilepsy Management

The classical ketogenic diet originated as a treatment for epilepsy, and remains an effective medical nutrition therapy for drug-resistant seizure disorders like Dravet Syndrome. For epilepsy, the diet is implemented carefully in a clinic setting, with ketogenic ratios of fats to carbs/protein of 3:1 or 4:1. Often shakes, liquids, and tube feeding provide sustenance.

Potential Applications for Depression

Small studies have explored using ketogenic diets as an intervention for major depressive disorder. It is postulated that keto may increase serotonin synthesis and BDNF, in the brain. Results thus far show a significant reduction in depression scores, after following a keto diet for several weeks. But sample sizes remain small, and larger randomized trials are warranted, to further investigate.

Implementing Keto to Prepare for Weight Loss Surgery

A very low-calorie, ketogenic diet is sometimes prescribed pre-surgery for morbid obesity, to shrink liver volume and visceral fat, allowing safer surgical access. This liquid formulation helps potentiate rapid and safe weight loss, before bariatric procedures. Close medical supervision is still required for nutrition status and medication adjustments, during keto-adaptation.

Mental Clarity and Focus on Keto

By providing an efficient alternative brain fuel in ketones and stabilizing energy, keto diets are reported to enhance many aspects of cognition and mental performance. Studies demonstrate improved memory, clarity, and ability to focus during ketosis. Ketones may also provide neuroprotective benefits. Further study of keto's effects on brain health is warranted.

Importance of Nutrient Density on Keto

On keto, daily food choices should maximize nutrient density, as overall intake volume is reduced. Prioritizing non-starchy vegetables, nuts, seeds, eggs, wild-caught fish, grass-fed meats, oils, and low-sugar fruits, ensures micronutrient needs are met. Supplementing with magnesium, potassium, calcium, zinc, and vitamin D, also helps prevent deficiencies when restricting food groups.

Using Keto for Polycystic Ovary Syndrome

Polycystic ovary syndrome (PCOS) involves metabolic dysfunction. Insulin resistance drives hormonal imbalances and ovarian cysts. Research indicates that lower carb, ketogenic diets can significantly improve PCOS, by enhancing insulin sensitivity, promoting ovulation and fertility, and aiding weight loss. This reduces key PCOS symptoms, like excess hair growth, acne, and absent periods.

47

Chapter 3
Starting Your Keto Journey

The journey of a thousand miles begins with a single step, so said Lao Tzu. As you stand on the brink of your keto journey, you may find the road ahead both exciting and a little daunting. The ketogenic diet, though significantly different from the traditional dietary norms, offers an array of potential health benefits. Still, making a lifestyle change is not always straightforward. It requires determination, patience, and most importantly, knowledge.

The purpose of this chapter, "Starting Your Keto Journey," is to provide you with the necessary information and tools, to help you navigate the early stages of transitioning to a ketogenic diet. From setting realistic expectations and preparing your pantry, to understanding the importance of tracking your progress and managing potential side effects, we've got you covered.

Change is not easy, but with the right guidance, it's certainly achievable. The first few steps of this new dietary path will be the most challenging, but once you start seeing and feeling the results, you'll realize it's worth it. This chapter is designed to be your trusted companion, providing step-by-step guidance to ensure your keto journey starts on the right foot.

So, take a deep breath, and let's embark on this exciting journey together!

1. Setting Realistic Expectations

Before embarking on your keto journey, it's important to set realistic expectations. This is not a magic pill that will solve all health issues overnight. It's a lifestyle change, and like all changes, it requires time. Weight loss, improved energy levels, better mental clarity - all these benefits will come, but not instantaneously.

Remember, everyone's body is different. How quickly you enter ketosis, the rate at which you lose weight, and how you feel overall will vary. Listen to your body, make adjustments as needed, and don't compare your journey with others. Patience and consistency will be your best friends on this journey.

2. Getting Your Pantry Ready

Start your keto journey by preparing your kitchen. Remove all high-carb and processed foods from your pantry and fridge. This includes pastas, bread, sugary cereals, cookies, candy, soda, and even certain fruits and vegetables. Remember, the statement, "out of sight, out of mind," is completely true.

Once you've cleared your kitchen of these items, it's time to restock with keto-friendly foods. Essential items include:

Healthy Fats: Extra virgin olive oil, coconut oil, grass-fed butter, avocado oil
Proteins: Grass-fed beef, free-range poultry, fatty fish, eggs
Low-Carb Vegetables: Leafy greens, broccoli, bell peppers, zucchini
Low-Glycemic Fruits: Berries, avocado, tomatoes
Dairy: Cheese, heavy cream, Greek yogurt (in moderation)
Nuts and Seeds: Almonds, walnuts, flaxseeds, chia seeds
Condiments: Mustard, apple cider vinegar, unsweetened ketchup, mayo
Sweeteners: Erythritol, stevia, monk fruit
Having a kitchen filled with these foods will make it much easier to stick to your new eating plan.

3. Learning to Calculate Your Macros

Macronutrients, or macros, are the nutrients your body needs in large amounts, namely carbohydrates, protein, and fats. When following a ketogenic diet, it's essential to understand how to calculate your macros. Here's a general guideline:

Carbohydrates: 5-10% of daily calories
Proteins: 20-25% of daily calories
Fats: 70-75% of daily calories

You can use online calculators to help determine your macros based on your age, sex, weight, activity level, and goals. It's important to note that these percentages aren't set in stone. Some people may need more protein, while others might need to adjust their fat intake. Listen to your body, and make adjustments as needed.

4. Meal Planning and Prepping

Meal planning and prepping can be your secret weapon for success on the ketogenic diet. Taking time each week to plan your meals and doing some prep work can save time, reduce stress, and help keep you on track. This can be as simple as jotting down your meals for the week, shopping for all your ingredients, and prepping some components ahead of time.

Don't be afraid to keep things simple, especially in the beginning. Stick with meals that you know and enjoy, simply adapting them to fit your new lifestyle. There are countless keto recipes available online

5. Understanding the Keto Flu and How to Mitigate It

When you first start a ketogenic diet, you may experience a group of symptoms commonly referred to as the "keto flu". These may include headaches, fatigue, irritability, nausea, and difficulty concentrating. The keto flu isn't an actual flu, but rather a group of symptoms that can occur as your body adapts to a drastic reduction in carbohydrate intake.

You can minimize the impact of the keto flu by staying hydrated, getting plenty of sleep, replenishing electrolytes, and gradually reducing your carb intake rather than going cold turkey.

6. The Importance of Hydration and Electrolytes

As your body transitions into ketosis, you'll likely notice an increase in urination. This is due to the diuretic effect of ketosis, which can cause you to lose electrolytes at a faster rate. Electrolytes are minerals that carry an electric charge and play a crucial role in maintaining fluid balance, nerve conduction, muscle contractions, and more.

To avoid electrolyte imbalances, be sure to consume plenty of fluids and foods rich in sodium, potassium, and magnesium. Additionally, you may consider an electrolyte supplement, particularly during the first few weeks of your keto transition.

7. Monitoring Your Progress

Keep track of your progress. This doesn't mean you should obsess over the scale, but regular check-ins can be motivating and help you identify areas that might need adjustment. You might track your weight, body measurements, energy levels, sleep quality, and cognitive improvements. Alternatively, you can use tools like ketone test strips or a blood ketone meter to measure your ketone levels, ensuring you're staying in ketosis.

8. Don't Fear the Fat, But Don't Overdo It

One of the common mistakes beginners make on a ketogenic diet is not consuming enough fat. Since fat is your primary source of energy on this diet, it's crucial to get enough of it. However, this doesn't mean you should gorge on unhealthy fats or exceed your daily caloric needs with fat alone. Remember, the goal is a well-balanced, nutrient-dense diet that puts your body into a state of ketosis.

9. Exercising on a Ketogenic Diet

Regular exercise is a crucial part of any healthy lifestyle, including a ketogenic lifestyle. When first starting your keto journey, you might find your exercise performance slightly decreased. Don't worry, as your body becomes adapted to burning fat for fuel, your performance will start to improve again.

Remember, the type of exercise you do can also impact your macronutrient needs. For instance, if you're doing heavy weightlifting or high-intensity interval training, you might need to increase your protein intake to support muscle recovery and growth.

10. Listening to Your Body

While it's important to have guidelines and rules to follow, it's equally crucial to listen to your body. If you're feeling hungry, eat. If you're feeling tired, rest. Your body is a sophisticated system that often knows what it needs. As you embark on your keto journey, cultivate an attitude of mindfulness, paying close attention to the signals your body sends you.

11. Socializing and Eating Out on a Keto Diet

One of the challenges people often face when transitioning to a ketogenic diet is dealing with social occasions or eating out. Fortunately, with a little planning and strategizing, you can maintain your diet and still enjoy these situations. When eating out, opt for dishes that are rich in protein and healthy fats, like grilled chicken or fish, and substitute starchy sides with non-starchy vegetables. Most restaurants are accommodating of dietary needs.

Social events can be a bit more challenging, especially if you're unsure what food will be available. Consider eating something before you go, or bring a keto-friendly dish to share. Remember, it's okay to kindly decline food that doesn't align with your dietary goals. Staying committed to your health is not rude, it's commendable.

12. Embracing the Learning Curve

Remember, there is a learning curve when starting a new diet, and the ketogenic diet is no different. You're likely to make mistakes, and that's okay. What's important is that you learn from them and continue to make progress. Be patient with yourself and remember why you started this journey in the first place.

13. Connecting with a Supportive Community

Having a support system can significantly improve your success on the ketogenic diet. Whether it's family, friends, or online communities, having people who understand and support your journey can be incredibly beneficial. Share your experiences, ask questions, and learn from others who are on the same path. You're not alone in this journey, and the shared wisdom of others can be a potent tool.

14. Continuing Education

Just because you've started your journey doesn't mean you should stop learning about the ketogenic diet. There's always more to learn, and continuing to educate yourself can help you make more informed decisions and better troubleshoot any issues that may arise. Listen to podcasts, read books, follow leading experts in the field - the more you know, the better equipped you'll be.

15. The Importance of Self-care

While diet is a critical component of health, it's not the only one. Don't forget to take care of your other needs as well. Get plenty of quality sleep, manage stress through practices like meditation or yoga, and engage in activities that bring you joy. Health isn't just about the food we eat; it's about the overall care we provide to our body, mind, and spirit.

16. Remembering the Importance of Fiber

Even though you're cutting back on carbs, you still need to make sure you're getting enough fiber. Fiber aids digestion, helps to keep you feeling full, and can also support gut health. Include plenty of low-carb, high-fiber vegetables in your diet, along with nuts and seeds.

17. Persistence is Key

Transitioning to a ketogenic lifestyle is a marathon, not a sprint. It requires consistency and commitment. There may be days when you struggle, and that's okay. What's important is that you don't give up. Keep your eye on your long-term health goals, and remember why you started.

18. Integrating Intermittent Fasting

Intermittent fasting (IF) is an eating pattern where you cycle between periods of eating and fasting. It's not about what foods to eat, but when you should eat them. Combining the ketogenic diet with IF can be powerful in reaching your health goals faster. This is because your body is already in fat-burning mode due to the low-carb intake, and IF can further enhance this effect.

Common methods include the 16/8 method (16 hours of fasting and an 8-hour eating window), the 5:2 diet (eating normally 5 days a week, reducing calories to 500-600 on two days), or eat-stop-eat (one or two 24-hour fasts per week). Before starting IF, it's recommended to consult with a healthcare provider, especially for those with medical conditions or who are pregnant.

19. Recognizing the Role of Stress and Sleep

Diet is just one piece of the health puzzle. High-stress levels and lack of sleep can hinder your keto progress. Chronic stress can lead to hormonal imbalances that may stall weight loss and even lead to weight gain. Likewise, sleep deprivation can mess with your hunger hormones, leading to increased appetite and cravings.

Practice good sleep hygiene by creating a dark, cool sleeping environment, and sticking to a regular sleep schedule. Also, engage in stress-reducing activities such as yoga, meditation, walks in nature, or reading a book.

20. Exploring Keto Variations

If the standard ketogenic diet feels too restrictive, know that there are other variations that you could explore:

Targeted Ketogenic Diet (TKD): This variation allows you to add carbs around workouts.
Cyclical Ketogenic Diet (CKD): A second variation involves periods of higher-carb refeeds, such as five ketogenic days followed by two high-carb days.
High-Protein Ketogenic Diet: This one is similar to standard ketogenic diet, but includes more protein The ratio is often 60% fat, 35% protein, and 5% carbs.
Remember, it's about finding a sustainable approach that fits your lifestyle, preferences, and health goals.

21. Understanding the Role of Supplements

While it's best to get your nutrients from food, some supplements can be beneficial on a ketogenic diet. These might include:

MCT Oil: This can be added to drinks for a boost in ketone levels.

Exogenous Ketones: These increase the ketone levels in your body, mimicking ketosis.

Electrolytes: These help to prevent mineral imbalances.

Fiber: Prevent constipation by eating more fiber.

Omega-3 Fatty Acids: They support heart health.

Before starting any supplement regimen, it's advisable to consult a healthcare provider.

22. Enjoying the Journey

Finally, remember to enjoy the journey! While reaching your goals is important, it's equally vital to enjoy the process. Celebrate your wins, learn from your challenges, and keep exploring what feels best for your body. It's not about perfection, but progress and wellness. Keep an open mind, be kind to yourself, and remember - you've got this!

23. Navigating Common Pitfalls

Like any new endeavor, the keto journey can come with its share of pitfalls. Let's discuss some of these common traps and how to avoid them:

Going Too Fast: One common mistake is drastically reducing your carb intake overnight. This abrupt change can result in severe keto flu symptoms and make you want to give up. It's often better to slowly lower your carb intake over a few weeks to allow your body to adjust.

Neglecting Veggie Intake: While it's true that some vegetables contain carbs, many are high in fiber and thus low in net carbs. Plus, they are packed with vital nutrients and antioxidants. Don't make the mistake of avoiding vegetables on keto; instead, opt for nutrient-rich, low-carb options like leafy greens, broccoli, and zucchini.

Not Getting Enough Sleep: Lack of sleep can interfere with weight loss and overall health. Try to get 7–9 hours of quality sleep per night.

24. Recalibrating Your Keto Approach As Needed

Remember that the ketogenic diet is not a one-size-fits-all solution. Your ideal macronutrient breakdown, caloric intake, and even the types of food you eat may vary, based on factors like your age, gender, activity level, and specific health goals. Don't be afraid to adjust and experiment to find what works best for you.

25. Expanding Your Keto Recipe Repertoire

One key to long-term keto success is keeping your meals interesting and tasty. Fortunately, there are countless keto-friendly recipes available for every meal, snack, and even dessert. Exploring these recipes can help prevent food boredom and keep you motivated and excited about your ketogenic lifestyle.

26. Preparing for Plateaus

Almost everyone hits a plateau at some point on their keto journey. This is a period where, despite your best efforts, your progress seems to stall. When this happens, it's important not to get discouraged. Instead, see it as an opportunity to reassess and make any necessary adjustments to your diet, exercise routine, sleep schedule, or stress management practices.

27. Prioritizing Whole Foods

While there are plenty of keto-friendly processed products on the market, try to make whole, unprocessed foods the foundation of your diet. These foods are typically more nutrient-dense and free from the added sugars and unhealthy fats that can be found in many processed products.

And remember, the journey towards a healthier, keto-adapted you, is a marathon, not a sprint. Be patient with yourself, celebrate the progress you've made, and don't lose sight of why you started this journey. You're not just transforming your diet; you're transforming your life. You're proving that you have the power to take control of your health and well-being, one keto-adapted day at a time. With every choice you make, every challenge you overcome, you're becoming a stronger, healthier, more confident version of yourself. That's something worth celebrating!

The number on the scale is not always the best measure of keto success. Things like improved body composition, increased energy levels, better lab results and reduced inflammation matter too. An important part of sticking to the keto diet is to track metrics beyond just the numbers on the scale. Take monthly progress photos to examine changes in body shape. Use a measuring tape to track inches lost from your waist, hips, arms and thighs. Log non-scale victories, like better sleep quality, improved mood or increased mental focus, that often come with ketogenic eating. Get blood work done occasionally to monitor internal improvements. Record how your clothes are fitting as you lose weight. Consider all these markers, equally important signs of progress, not just the weight on the scale.

Hitting a weight loss plateau while following the ketogenic diet can be frustrating, but there are ways to troubleshoot stalled progress. First, re-calculate your macros and calorie intake to ensure you're eating at an appropriate deficit for your stats. Next, consider intermittent fasting, which can help stimulate renewed fat burn during a plateau. Also, check for hidden carb sources like sauces, dressings or low-carb treats that may be kicking you out of ketosis. Cutting these out can help break the stall. Finally, be patient and trust the process - your weight will likely begin dropping again soon with a little troubleshooting. Another tip to help push through a stall is increasing exercise, especially strength training, to build metabolism-boosting muscle. Cutting back on dairy products can help, since dairy can stimulate insulin. Reduce unhealthy fats and boost healthy fats like olive oil and avocado. Consider a brief "fat fast" where you consume about 1,000 calories per day from only healthy fats, to jumpstart weight loss. Drink more water to flush out retaining water weight. Manage stress via yoga, meditation, massage, etc. since high cortisol inhibits weight loss. With a little diligence, you can break through plateaus.

Carefully reading nutrition labels is crucial for keto success. Look first at the serving size and carbohydrate count. Net carbs (total carbs minus fiber and sugar alcohols) should be low to fit into your daily limit. Also check calories, protein content, and types of fat. The ingredients list ideally should be short and contain recognizable whole foods. Watch for sneaky sources of added sugars. Comparing several products helps identify the best options for your carb and macronutrient needs. Reading labels, soon becomes second nature. Taking a few extra minutes to analyze nutritional information can be an empowering part of your keto success.

Eating keto when dining out requires strategy, especially at the start. To avoid pitfalls, don't arrive starving - have a small snack beforehand, so you don't dive into the bread basket. Peruse the menu online first when possible, and pick your meal in advance. Stick to simple proteins that are grilled, baked, or broiled. Ask for non-starchy vegetables instead of high-carb sides. Request sauces and dressings on the side to control portions, and skip sugary cocktails, desserts, and anything breaded or fried. Staying keto through indulgent work dinners or celebratory meals, is possible with a little preparation and willpower. Being selective sets you up for success.

With savvy shopping, the ketogenic diet doesn't have to be expensive. Focus on affordable proteins like eggs, whole chickens, pork, canned fish, and tougher, fattier cuts of beef to save money. Buy frozen vegetables when they are on sale. Stick to less costly nuts, like peanuts and almonds, in bulk. Purchase olive and avocado oils in large containers. Supplement meals with low-cost pantry staples like broths, spices, and condiments. Plan meals based on what's currently on sale or in season. Cook at home in bulk, and use leftovers the next day. With a little effort, creativity, and strategic planning, keto foods can fit most budgets.

On keto, certain micronutrients require a little extra attention to avoid potential shortfalls. Make sure you are getting adequate magnesium, which is essential for regulating blood sugar, aiding sleep, and reducing muscle cramps. Eat plenty of leafy greens, nuts, and seeds and supplement if needed. Get enough sodium, potassium and phosphorus by focusing on electrolyte-rich, whole foods and proper hydration. Don't neglect fiber from sources like low-carb vegetables, berries, nuts, and seeds. Include vitamin C-rich foods like bell peppers, citrus fruits, tomatoes and broccoli. Incorporate calcium via sardines, canned fish with bones, and hard, low-carb dairy, like cheese. Eat more eggs, meat, fish, and shellfish for zinc and B vitamins. With sound nutrition principles, keto diets can be nutritionally balanced and complete. The key is targeting a wide variety of micronutrient-dense, whole foods.

Sophia Ramos

Chapter 4
Essential Kitchen Setup for Keto

Introduction

Transitioning into a ketogenic lifestyle, requires more than just an understanding of the diet and its benefits. It also requires a change in your kitchen - your sanctuary for creating nourishing, keto-friendly meals. This chapter will delve into how to set up your kitchen, what foods to stock up on, what kitchen gadgets might come in handy, and tips to manage your kitchen for easy, efficient, meal prep.

1. Cleaning out the Pantry

The first step in setting up your keto kitchen is cleaning out your pantry. This process can be liberating, but may also feel overwhelming, especially if you have a lot of non-keto items. Start by removing all high-carb items, including bread, pasta, rice, beans, sugary snacks, cereals, and baking supplies like flour and sugar.

2. Keto-Friendly Pantry Staples

Once your pantry is cleared out, it's time to restock it with keto-friendly staples. Here are some items to consider:

Oils and Fats: Extra virgin olive oil, coconut oil, avocado oil, and grass-fed butter or ghee, are all excellent choices. Remember, healthy fats are the cornerstone of a keto diet.

Nuts and Seeds: Almonds, macadamias, walnuts, flaxseeds, chia seeds, and pumpkin seeds are all low in carbs and high in healthy fats. Just remember to monitor portion sizes, as carbs can add up.

Canned Goods: Tuna, sardines, and salmon are excellent for quick meals. Also, consider stocking up on canned vegetables for emergencies.

Low-carb Flours: Almond flour and coconut flour are great for low-carb baking.

Sweeteners: Erythritol, stevia, monk fruit, and allulose are popular sugar substitutes on keto.

Spices: Spices can add a lot of flavor to your meals without adding carbs. Stock up on your favorites, and don't be afraid to try new ones!

3. The Keto Fridge

Next, it's time to arrange your refrigerator. Fresh vegetables, dairy, eggs, and meats are all staple items on a keto diet:

Vegetables: Leafy greens, broccoli, cauliflower, zucchini, bell peppers, and avocados are all excellent choices.

Dairy: Cheese, cream, Greek yogurt, and butter are all keto-friendly. Opt for full-fat versions wherever possible.

Proteins: Eggs, beef, poultry, pork, and fish are key sources of protein on a ketogenic diet.

4. Freezer Essentials

Your freezer can be a lifesaver for storing meats, seafood, and frozen vegetables. It's also a great place to store batch-cooked meals or leftovers for those busy days when cooking is not an option.

5. Keto-Friendly Beverages

Stay hydrated with water, herbal teas, bone broth, and coffee or tea. Avoid sugary beverages, including most fruit juices and soft drinks.

6. Meal Prep and Planning

Meal prepping is a game-changer for sticking to your keto diet. By dedicating a few hours a week to prepare meals, you can save time, reduce stress, and stay on track with your keto goals. Consider investing in quality containers for storage. Glass containers are a versatile and environmentally-friendly choice.

7. Essential Keto Kitchen Tools

Having the right kitchen tools can make cooking easier and more enjoyable. While everyone's preferences and needs may differ, here are some commonly used tools in a keto kitchen:

Food Processor: Ideal for making cauliflower rice, blending sauces, or chopping nuts.

Spiralizer: Great for making zucchini noodles or other vegetable "pasta."
Blender: Essential for making smoothies, puréed soups, or bulletproof coffee.

Slow Cooker or Instant Pot: These appliances can be a lifesaver for busy people, allowing you to cook in bulk, with minimal effort.

Kitchen Scale: This can be especially useful in the beginning as you familiarize yourself with portion sizes.

8. Organizing Your Kitchen

An organized kitchen can significantly streamline your meal prep and cooking process. Try these tips:

Keep your counters as clutter-free as possible. This gives you more space to prepare your meals and makes cleaning easier.

Store your most-used items within easy reach. This might be your favorite spices, cooking utensils, or pots and pans.

Label your pantry items, especially if you're using unfamiliar ingredients like different low-carb flours or sweeteners.

Regularly clean out your fridge and pantry to avoid wasting food. Make sure to use up fresh produce before it spoils, and keep an eye on the expiration dates of your pantry items.

9. Batch Cooking and Freezing

One of the keys to success on a ketogenic diet is having keto-friendly meals readily available. That's where batch cooking comes in handy.. By cooking large quantities of a meal and freezing it in individual portions, you'll have ready-to-eat meals for busy days. Soups, stews, casseroles, and slow cooker meals are all excellent candidates for batch cooking.

10. Snacks on the Go

One challenging aspect of any diet can be finding suitable snacks, especially when you're out and about. Preparing keto-friendly snacks can help you avoid temptation. Consider options like hard-boiled eggs, cheese sticks, nuts, seeds, or homemade keto bars.

11. Mastering Keto Substitutes

Part of the fun (and the challenge) of a ketogenic diet is finding low-carb substitutes for your favorite high-carb foods. From cauliflower rice to almond flour bread to zucchini noodles, the possibilities are endless. Having these substitutes in your repertoire can make sticking to your keto diet more enjoyable and sustainable.

12. Keto Baking Essentials

If you love baking, you'll be glad to know you can still enjoy this pastime on a keto diet. Stock up on almond flour, coconut flour, unsweetened cocoa powder, low-carb sweeteners, and xanthan gum for binding. From brownies to cheesecake to bread, there are plenty of delicious keto baking recipes to try.

13. Cooking with Keto Fats

Understanding how and when to use different fats and oils can enhance your keto cooking. For instance, avocado oil and refined coconut oil have a high smoke point, making them suitable for high-heat cooking. In contrast, extra virgin olive oil is best for low-heat cooking or for drizzling on finished dishes.

14. Hydrating Right

Staying well-hydrated is important on a keto diet. Keep a water bottle handy at all times. Don't forget, you can also hydrate with beverages like herbal tea and bone broth.

Setting up your kitchen for keto may seem like a daunting task, but taking it step by step can make the process manageable and even fun. Remember, the effort you put into preparing your kitchen and learning new ways of cooking and eating, is an investment in your health and well-being. Happy cooking!

15. Exploring Keto-Friendly Condiments

Your kitchen isn't complete without a range of flavorful condiments to enhance your meals. Many condiments are high in added sugars, but there are plenty of keto-friendly alternatives:

Mayonnaise: Ideal for salads and dips. Look for versions made with healthy oils like avocado oil

Mustard: Adds a tangy kick to your meals without adding carbs

Hot Sauce: A great way to spice up your dishes
(Just check the label to ensure there's no added sugar.)

Vinegar: Balsamic, apple cider, white wine, and red wine vinegar, can all add depth to your dishes. Be mindful of balsamic vinegar, as it can contain more carbs.

Soy Sauce or Tamari: This adds an Asian flair to your dishes. Opt for gluten-free versions if you're avoiding gluten.

Sugar-Free Ketchup: Regular ketchup is high in sugar, but there are sugar-free versions available.

16. Practical Tips for Keto Grocery Shopping

Grocery shopping for a new diet can be challenging. Here are some tips to make it easier:

Plan Ahead: Before you head to the grocery store, make a meal plan for the week. From there, you can create a detailed shopping list of what you'll need.

Shop the Perimeter: The freshest, most natural foods are usually located around the perimeter of the store. This is where you'll find fresh fruits and vegetables, meats, and dairy products.

Read Labels: Just because something is labeled as "low-carb" doesn't necessarily mean it's keto-friendly. Be sure to read the nutrition facts and ingredient list to ensure it fits within your keto macros.

Buy in Bulk: Non-perishable items, like nuts, seeds, and certain canned goods, can often be bought in bulk to save money.

17. Navigating Dining Out and Social Events

While most of your meals will likely be home-cooked, it's important to know how to stick to your keto diet when dining out or attending social events. Research the restaurant's menu ahead of time, look for meat- or fish-based dishes, ask for substitutions (like veggies instead of a side of potatoes), and don't be afraid to ask questions about the preparation of the dishes.

18. Developing Your Keto Cooking Skills

As with any diet, variety is key to sticking with it. This might mean stepping out of your comfort zone and expanding your cooking skills. Try new recipes, experiment with different spices and flavors, and don't be afraid of making mistakes. The more you cook, the more you'll improve.

19. Keeping Your Kitchen Keto-Friendly Over Time

Maintaining a keto-friendly kitchen is an ongoing process. You might find new foods or ingredients that you love, or new recipes that require different tools. You'll also need to periodically reassess your pantry and fridge to make sure they're still serving your needs. Over time, your kitchen will continue to evolve, along with your journey on the ketogenic diet.

20. A Kitchen That Supports Your Goals

Ultimately, your kitchen should support your goals. This might mean different things to different people. For some, it might mean having a variety of quick, easy meal options on hand. For others, it might mean having the tools and ingredients to experiment with more complex keto recipes. Whatever it means to you, remember that your kitchen is a key player in your keto journey.

Remember that a keto kitchen is not just about the foods you eat, but also the way you prepare and think about food. It's about making conscious choices that support your health and well-being. It might take some time to fully transition your kitchen to a keto-friendly space, but it's worth the effort. With the right setup, you'll be well-equipped to enjoy the keto lifestyle for the long term.

Stocking your fridge and pantry properly is key to keto success. Having the right foods on hand means you'll always have quick, easy meal and snack options available. Fill your fridge with eggs, raw nuts, nut butters, full-fat cheese, coconut milk or heavy cream, olives, avocados, leafy greens, cruciferous veggies, like broccoli and cauliflower, fresh berries, coconut yogurt, leftover meat, fish, chicken, and pre-prepped veggies for snacks. Your freezer should contain meat, poultry, fish, berries, and veggies, like cauliflower rice and zucchini noodles. Frozen items are great for quick meals when you don't have time to prep. Your pantry should be stocked with canned fish like salmon and sardines, oils like olive oil and avocado oil, nuts and seeds, nut and seed butters, nutritional yeast, spices, sugars like monk fruit and erythritol, teas and coffee, nut flours, baking basics like baking powder and xanthan gum, vinegar, mustards, olives, and shelf-stable, full-fat coconut milk. A properly stocked fridge and pantry means you'll always have access to quick breakfasts like eggs, avocado toast, or chia pudding. It provides easy lunch options like tuna salad wrapped in lettuce leaves or leftovers reheated. And it offers the ingredients to whip up simple dinners like fajita skillets, sheet pan chicken and veggies, or salmon with pesto zucchini noodles.

When buying fresh produce on keto, go for variety, quality, and nutrient density. You should aim for a diverse array of colorful veggies to ensure you'll get a wide range of vitamins, minerals, antioxidants, and phytonutrients. Target leafy greens, cruciferous vegetables, squash, zucchini, eggplant, mushrooms, asparagus, cucumbers, peppers, onions and tomatoes. Prioritize organic and local foods, whenever possible. For fruits, focus on lower carb options like berries, green apples, grapefruit, and small portions of stone fruits. Avoid high carb fruits like bananas, mangos, grapes, and pineapple. Don't be afraid of frozen produce, either! Frozen veggies and fruits are picked at peak ripeness and frozen immediately to lock in nutrients. You'll want to prioritize colorful options like raspberries, blueberries, mango, spinach, kale, and mixed veggies. Quality produce means better nutrition and texture. Inspect fruits and veggies and choose ones that are free of blemishes, bruising, or damage. Sturdier produce with tighter skins will store longer, while softer berries and leafy greens are more delicate, and best eaten within a few days of purchasing. Proper storage helps prolong freshness too.

Once you've nailed down the basics, consider branching out to more unique ingredients that add diversity and nutrients. Some keto-friendly, exotic items to try, include dragonfruit, guava, starfruit, passionfruit, lychee, shiitake mushrooms, oyster mushrooms, enoki mushrooms, maitake mushrooms, nori seaweed, wakame seaweed, kombu seaweed, basil, cilantro, parsley, mint, oregano, thyme, turmeric, cinnamon, cardamom, paprika, cumin, coriander, green tea, oolong tea, herbal tea blends, and nutritional yeast flakes, for a savory, cheesy flavor.Kalamata olives, castelvetrano olives, oil-cured olives, coconut aminos, sesame oil, and chili crisp sauce can add a zing to your already loved foods. Incorporating new flavors keeps your keto journey exciting. These items allow you to recreate ethnic dishes or add flair to staple meals. Start small by adding one new ingredient each week and playing around with simple recipes before working up to more complex cooking.

When purchasing meat, poultry, fish, and eggs on keto, quality is key for both health and taste reasons. You'll want to look for pasture-raised, grass-fed, and organic options whenever possible, to ensure more humane treatment of animals and better nutrition. Go for wild caught fish over farmed, since wild fish get more exercise, eat more natural diets, and are lower in contaminants. Opt for fattier cuts of meat like chicken thighs over breasts, since the fat makes them more moist and flavorful. Don't be afraid to try organ meats like liver or heart, since they are actually some of the most nutrient-dense cuts you can eat. For eggs, look for ones from pasture-raised hens, since their omega-3 content is higher. Check expiration dates and pick the freshest options available. With seafood, make sure it smells clean, not fishy. Eating high-quality proteins, provides more vitamins, minerals, and beneficial fats to optimize your health on keto.

Meal prepping can be a huge time saver that helps you stick to keto. It allows you to cook ahead in batches, so healthy meals are ready to grab and go. Dedicate a few hours on your day off for prepping and put on some music or a podcast, to make it enjoyable. Freeze pre-portioned meals in containers, so you always have a ready stash to defrost. Soups, stews, and chili, work great for freezing. Pre-chop veggies and store in containers for easy snacking, paired with tuna salad or hummus. Make egg muffins with your favorite keto veggies baked in, that will last 5–7 days refrigerated. Marinate proteins like chicken breasts in batches, so they are infused with lots of flavor. Cook extra meat, chicken, or fish, at dinner to use for lunches, paired with veggies. Make a big keto-friendly salad at the start of the week, and add different proteins and dressings each day. With strategic meal prep, you'll always have keto-friendly options available, when hunger strikes or life gets busy.

Cooking with quality fats is important on keto, both for health and flavor. Some of the top choices are extra virgin olive oil, coconut oil, avocado oil, butter or ghee, bacon grease, and tallow, or lard. Olive oil is extremely versatile with its high smoke point and delicious flavor. Use it for light sautéing or drizzling onto salads and dips. Coconut oil provides lauric acid and MCTs that are quickly metabolized, making it great for higher heat cooking. Try avocado oil for pan frying and stir fries, due to its high smoke point and mild flavor. Butter or ghee, impart richness and are ideal for low to moderate heat cooking. Bacon grease is great for sautéing veggies or eggs, but make sure to use homemade grease from high quality bacon. Animal fats, like tallow or lard, are very stable for high heat cooking as long as they come from pasture-raised animals. Using the right cooking fats not only optimizes health qualities but also enhances flavor and texture.

Having the proper kitchen tools makes keto cooking much easier and more enjoyable. Over time, invest in quality items, like a good chef's knife, cutting boards for separate meat and produce prep, stainless steel or enamel coated, cast iron skillets and saucepans, stainless steel or ceramic baking sheets and casserole dishes, a slow cooker for hands-off batch cooking, an immersion blender to purée soups and sauces in the pot, a spiralizer for turning veggies into noodle form, and a food processor to chop veggies, make cauliflower rice, blend dips and more. Having the right tools saves time in the kitchen and makes food prep and cooking much more efficient. Slowly build up your collection of quality kitchen tools over time.

Dining out while staying keto is very doable with some planning. Research the menu in advance and pick a protein-focused dish. Ask for any carb-heavy sides to be substituted with extra veggies. Request butter or olive oil instead of bread, before your meal. Skip breaded, fried appetizers, and order a salad instead. Stay away from sugary sauces and dressings, by asking for them on the side. For dessert, opt for fresh berries with whipped cream or dark chocolate. Don't be shy when it comes to asking your server questions about how foods are prepared and ingredients used. If your meal comes with multiple carb sides, ask to substitute extra veggies or a double salad instead. The key is knowing what to look for, asking the right questions, and not being afraid to make substitutions. With the right modifications, you can dine out anywhere on keto.

Salad bars can be a great option for keto-friendly lunches. Build your base with plenty of dark leafy greens like spinach, kale, or romaine. Pile on the veggies, like cucumbers, tomatoes, mushrooms, broccoli, cauliflower, peppers, and sprouts. Add protein with eggs, salmon, tuna, chicken, or ham slices. Cheese, olives, avocado, nuts, and seeds, incorporate healthy fats. Avoid prepared salads with sugary dressings, and instead opt for olive oil and vinegar, or lemon juice. Stay away from starchy sides like pasta salad, potato salad, rice, or beans. Fruit is fine in moderation, so stick to berries and melons versus pineapple, grapes, and mandarin oranges. With the right choices, salad bars can provide filling, nutrient-packed, keto meals easily.

Having keto-friendly snacks on hand helps curb cravings and prevents grabbing sugar-laden options when hunger hits. Always keep your kitchen stocked with tasty snacks like nuts including almonds, walnuts, pecans, and macadamia nuts. Keep a supply of seeds, including pumpkin, sunflower, and chia seeds. Natural nut butters without added sugars, avocado halves, hard-boiled eggs, leftover cooked meat rolled around cheese, veggies for dipping in guacamole or hummus, frozen berries with heavy cream, low-carb jerky or pemmican, and keto protein bars with minimal net carbs, are great to have on hand.Snack time should be satisfying, to bridge meals while remaining in ketosis. Smart snack choices make this possible.

Potlucks, barbecues, and other social gatherings with food, can be tricky to navigate on keto. But with the right strategies, you can still enjoy yourself, while sticking to your diet. Offer to bring a keto-friendly side dish or dessert, so you know there will be something you can eat, like a green salad, vegetable tray, or fresh fruit salad. Survey all the foods being offered first, before filling your plate, and stick to meat- or veggie-based dishes, while avoiding carb-laden options. Only take small spoonfuls of richer side dishes to balance your plate, and avoid pasta salads, potato dishes, rice, bread and sweet desserts. For beverages, stick with unsweetened iced tea, water, or mineral water with lemon/lime and avoid sugary sodas and juices. If it's a barbecue, fill your plate with burger patties, grilled proteins, and big servings of salad and veggies. With mindfulness and moderation, potlucks and BBQs can be enjoyed on the keto diet.

Weddings, work events, and parties require careful management of your keto eating, but with smart strategies, you can stick to your plan, while still enjoying special occasions. Research the catering menu ahead of time and note keto-friendly options - choose meat, fish, and veggie dishes. Ask about getting salads and vegetables without high-carb dressings and sauces, and request olive oil and vinegar instead. Unless you know they are low-carb, avoid the bread basket, dinner rolls, and bread-based appetizers. For appetizers, stick to veggie crudités, cheese and cured meat platters, shrimp cocktail, or oysters. Skip the pasta, rice, potato, and quinoa dishes. Load up on extra proteins and veggies instead.

For dessert, limit yourself to just a few bites of richer options like cheesecake and choose fresh berries as an alternative. Sip on dry wines, champagne, or spirits rather than beer, sweet wines, cocktails, and sugary sodas. With mindfulness and selectivity, you can navigate special occasion eating on keto successfully.

Alcohol can absolutely be enjoyed in moderation on a keto diet, as long as you stick to the lowest carbohydrate options. Good choices include dry wines, like red, white and sparkling, Brut champagne, in 6 ounce or less serving sizes., Dry spirits like whiskey, scotch, vodka, gin, and rum in 1-2 ounce servings per drink, diluted with soda water, are smart choices. Also, light beers and hard seltzers, under 3-4g net carbs, limited to 1-2 per day maximum, dry fortified wines like unsweetened sherries and ports in 2 ounces or less daily, cocktails like vodka soda, martini, Manhattan and old-fashioned are tasty examples of spirited drinks, and make sure to specify no sugary mixers or juices. The key is to keep servings moderate, avoiding high carb mixers, and tracking your carbohydrates. When in doubt, drink a spirit on the rocks with soda water and lime.

One tactic for keto success is recreating favorite comfort foods with low-carb ingredients. Get creative by coating breaded foods in crushed pork rinds or almond flour instead of flour based breading., Swapout pasta for zucchini noodles, hearts of palm, or shirataki noodle., Turn cauliflower, broccoli stems, and rutabaga into "rice", replace potatoes with turnips, radishes, jicama or eggplant, and use lettuce leaves, portobello caps, or cheese crisps, instead of bread. Make pizza crusts from almond flour, cheese, or eggplant, switch sugary soda to sparkling water with lemon/lime and zero-carb sweetener, and blend frozen avocado and cocoa powder with sweetener, for "nice cream" instead of ice cream. Make keto pancakes with almond flour, eggs, and a touch of sweetener. Being innovative with substitutions allows you to still enjoy all your favorite comfort foods on the keto diet.

It's normal to crave something sweet occasionally on keto. Healthier ways to indulge your sweet tooth include eating the right fruits, 90% dark chocolate, chia seed pudding, keto mug cakes, and yummy homemade frozen yogurt bites, with stevia and vanilla. Smoothies made with avocado, cacao powder, and sweetener, make a great afternoon snack, and homemade keto protein bars, or fat bombs, are easy to take when traveling. Desserts made with keto-approved sweeteners, like monk fruit or allulose, and creamy, blended, frozen coconut butter can be a nice addition to your day.The key is to keep portions small, and find ways to add richness and protein, which will naturally slow the blood sugar response, and keep cravings in check. These tips will help you satisfy sweet cravings, the smart way.

Investing in quality food storage containers, helps keep your keto foods fresh for meal prepping and saving leftovers. Look for BPA-free containers, to avoid chemicals leaching into food. Choose airtight containers that keep food fresh and prevent leakage. Opt for microwave and dishwasher safe products for easy use, and consider glass or stainless steel containers, for chemical safety. Get a variety of sizes like small containers for snacks and large ones for meal prepping. Keep in mind, nesting containers save storage space. Make sure lids match containers and seal tightly, and having the right food storage containers allows you to safely store and transport meals, leftovers, and snacks for your keto lifestyle.

Sticking to keto is tough if carb-laden temptations are lurking in your pantry and fridge. Do a sweep and remove pasta, rice, bread, crackers, baked goods, sugary snacks, like cookies, chips and candy, starchy vegetables like potatoes and sweet potatoes, beans, peas, lentils, sugary cereals, granola bars, oatmeal, fruit juices, sports drinks, soda, and condiments. Removing tempting items high in carbs, makes it much easier to stick to the keto diet, since those non-keto foods won't beckon you from the kitchen.

Sophia Ramos

Chapter 5

Keto-Friendly Grocery Shopping

A vital step in your keto journey is understanding how to grocery shop effectively. This chapter will guide you on how to fill your cart with keto-friendly items, read nutrition labels correctly, and navigate through the grocery store with confidence. Whether you're a novice or a seasoned shopper, these tips will help you make the best choices for your ketogenic diet.

1. Planning Your Shopping List

Before stepping foot in the grocery store, it's crucial to plan your shopping list. Base your list on your weekly meal plan, ensuring to cover all meals, snacks, and beverages. A well-planned shopping list not only saves time, but also helps to avoid impulse purchases, which may not be keto-friendly.

2. Shopping the Perimeter

Grocery stores are typically designed with fresh food items like vegetables, meats, and dairy along the perimeter, while processed foods are located in the middle aisles. Stick to the perimeter as much as possible, where you can find most of the whole foods for your keto diet.

3. Understanding Food Labels

Reading food labels is a vital skill for keto grocery shopping. Here's what to look for:

Carb Content: Check the total carbohydrates and the fiber content. You're interested in net carbs, which is total carbs minus fiber.

Ingredients: Look for natural, whole food ingredients, and avoid items with added sugars, unhealthy fats, and unnecessary additives.

Serving Size: Always check the serving size. Nutritional information is typically given per serving, not for the entire package.

4. Choosing High-Quality Fats

The keto diet is high in fats, but it's essential to choose high-quality, healthy fats. Look for sources like avocados, nuts and seeds, olives, fatty fish, and grass-fed meats. Avoid trans fats and limit your intake of refined vegetable oils.

5. Selecting Low-Carb Vegetables

Most of your carbs on a keto diet will come from vegetables. Focus on low-carb, non-starchy vegetables, such as leafy greens, broccoli, cauliflower, zucchini, bell peppers, and asparagus.

6. Picking the Right Proteins

Protein is an important part of a keto diet, but it's important not to overdo it, as excess protein can be converted into glucose in your body, taking you out of ketosis. Choose high-quality protein sources like grass-fed beef, free-range poultry, sustainable fish, and pasture-raised eggs.

7. Dairy on a Keto Diet

Full-fat dairy products are usually a good fit for a keto diet. They provide high-quality protein, essential vitamins, and healthy fats. Opt for products like full-fat Greek yogurt, heavy cream, butter, and a variety of cheeses.

8. Navigating the Snack Aisle

Snacking on a keto diet can be a challenge, especially when faced with the variety in the snack aisle. Look for low-carb snack options like nuts and seeds, cheese, and olives. Be wary of "low-carb" or "sugar-free" products, as they often contain hidden carbs or artificial ingredients.

9. Selecting Keto-Friendly Beverages

Water is the best beverage on a keto diet, but other options include unsweetened coffee and tea, mineral water, and bone broth. Be cautious with alcohol, as it can slow down weight loss and some alcoholic beverages can be high in carbs.

10. Frozen vs. Fresh Foods

While fresh is often best, frozen foods can be a convenient and nutritious option, especially when certain foods are out of season. Frozen low-carb vegetables, berries, and seafood are good choices.

11. Don't Forget About Condiments

Condiments can enhance the flavor of your meals, but many store-bought versions are loaded with sugar. Look for sugar-free or low-carb options, or consider making your own. Keto-friendly condiments include mayonnaise, mustard, full-fat salad dressings, vinegar, hot sauce, and sugar-free ketchup.

12. The Power of Herbs and Spices

Herbs and spices not only enhance the taste of your food, but they also come with numerous health benefits. They are also generally low in carbs. Stock up on a variety of herbs and spices like oregano, basil, thyme, rosemary, turmeric, cumin, chili powder, cinnamon, and more.

13. Nuts and Seeds

Nuts and seeds are a great source of healthy fats and protein. They can be eaten as a snack, used in baking, or added to salads and other dishes for extra crunch. Opt for raw or dry-roasted versions, and avoid those coated with sugars or vegetable oils. Some of the most keto-friendly options include macadamia nuts, pecans, almonds, walnuts, flax seeds, chia seeds, and pumpkin seeds.

14. Be Aware of Hidden Sugars

There are many different names for sugar, and food manufacturers often use this to their advantage. Be on the lookout for words like dextrose, fructose, sucrose, maltose, corn syrup, maltodextrin, and others. Even foods that seem healthy can contain hidden sugars.

15. Shopping for Keto Baking

Baking on a ketogenic diet is possible, but it requires some unique ingredients. Almond flour and coconut flour are excellent low-carb substitutes for wheat flour. Erythritol, stevia, and monk fruit are natural sweeteners that have no effect on blood sugar levels.

16. Preparing for the Unexpected

It's always a good idea to have some quick and easy keto-friendly options on hand for those times when you need a meal in a pinch. Things like canned tuna or salmon, eggs, pre-cooked meats, frozen vegetables, and full-fat cheese can all be lifesavers.

17. Remember Hydration

Staying hydrated is crucial on a keto diet, as the diet has a diuretic effect. Be sure to drink plenty of water throughout the day. Electrolyte supplements or broths can also be beneficial, especially in the beginning stages of the diet, when the risk of "keto flu" is higher.

18. Don't Forget About Offal

While it may not be as popular or as palatable to some, organ meats are incredibly nutrient-dense and can be a great addition to a ketogenic diet. Liver, kidney, heart - these are all rich in vitamins and minerals and are typically cheaper than other cuts of meat.

19. The Importance of Variety

Eating a varied diet is important for getting a range of nutrients and for keeping meals exciting. Try to incorporate a range of different meats, fish, vegetables, nuts, seeds, and dairy products into your diet.

20. Shopping Online

For hard-to-find items, consider shopping online. There are many online grocery stores that offer a wide variety of ketogenic foods that you might not find in your local store.

Keto-friendly grocery shopping doesn't have to be daunting. With a little planning and knowledge, you'll be able to navigate the store with ease and fill your cart with delicious, healthy, and satisfying foods that support your ketogenic lifestyle.

21. Portion Control and Meal Prep

While shopping, it's crucial to keep in mind your portion sizes. Even keto-friendly foods can lead to weight gain, if eaten in excess. Invest in a kitchen scale, measuring cups, and spoons, to ensure you're adhering to your meal plan accurately. Also, consider buying food containers for meal prepping. Preparing your meals in advance saves time and ensures you always have a keto-friendly option ready.

22. Keeping Keto on a Budget

Sticking to a ketogenic diet doesn't have to be expensive. Here are a few tips to keep your grocery bills in check:

Buy in Bulk: Purchasing food in larger quantities often results in cost savings. Items like nuts, seeds, and certain meats can be bought in bulk and stored for long periods.

Eat Seasonally: Fruits and vegetables are generally cheaper when they're in season. Plus, they taste better too!

Don't Shy Away from Frozen: Frozen vegetables and fruits are often cheaper than fresh ones, and they're just as nutritious.

Meal Plan: Planning your meals helps prevent food waste, which in turn, saves money.

23. The Impact of a Keto Diet on Environment

The foods you choose not only impact your health but also the health of our planet. Opt for sustainably sourced seafood, pasture-raised poultry, and grass-fed meats whenever possible. Shopping local farmers' markets can also reduce the carbon footprint.

24. Exploring International Foods

Don't be afraid to explore the international aisle at your grocery store. Many cultures around the world naturally eat low-carb, and you can find inspiration for new dishes. Spices, sauces, and unique vegetables, can add exciting variety to your keto meals.

25. Cooking Oils and Fats

Choose your cooking oils carefully, as some are more suited to the high-fat keto diet than others. Extra virgin olive oil, coconut oil, and avocado oil are great for keto, as they're high in healthy monounsaturated and saturated fats. For high-heat cooking, choose oils with high smoke points, such as avocado oil.

26. Navigating the Seafood Section

Seafood is a fantastic source of protein and omega-3 fatty acids. Wild-caught fish is usually a better choice than farmed, as it's often higher in nutrients and lower in pollutants. Fatty fish like salmon, mackerel, and sardines, are especially good choices for keto.

27. Keto and Vegetarianism/Veganism

It's entirely possible to follow a keto diet while being vegetarian or even vegan. In these cases, your protein sources will be things like tempeh, tofu, seitan, and certain legumes (in moderation). For fats, focus on avocados, nuts and seeds, and high-quality plant oils.

28. The Allure of Convenience Foods

While it's perfectly fine to enjoy keto-friendly convenience foods from time to time, they shouldn't make up the bulk of your diet. Many are highly processed and contain additives and preservatives. They can be useful in a pinch, but aim for whole foods most of the time.

29. Making the Most of Your Grocery Trips

Regular grocery shopping can be a chore for some, but try to view it as an opportunity. It's your chance to make decisions that will shape your health, experiment with new foods and flavors, and ultimately invest in yourself.

With this comprehensive guide to keto-friendly grocery shopping, you are now prepared to make smart, keto-aligned choices that will support your dietary goals and enhance your overall health. It's not just about shopping; it's about adopting a new lifestyle and embracing healthier habits. As we conclude this chapter on keto-friendly grocery shopping, it's important to reflect on the key lessons and strategies we've covered. Adopting a ketogenic diet is a significant lifestyle change that requires dedication, planning and adaptability. By thoughtfully stocking your kitchen and pantry with keto-compliant ingredients, you set yourself up for success and make adherence to the diet more convenient.

When embarking on keto grocery shopping, resist the urge to be overwhelmed. Take it one shopping trip at a time. Make a list and stick to the perimeter of the store where the whole, unprocessed foods are stocked. Become a label reader to identify hidden sugars and unnecessary additives. Seek out quality sources of proteins, healthy fats, and low-carb vegetables. Mitigate expenses by buying in bulk, freezing surplus produce, and awaiting sales on staple items.

It's wise to identify your personal triggers ahead of time. For some, the bakery section, with its aroma of fresh breads and pastries, is enough to derail willpower. Scope out the store layout, and make a plan to avoid temptation zones. Bringing a snack can help curb hunger pangs that lead to poor impulse purchases. If family members or roommates object, make sure to delineate separate shelves and storage areas.

As you adjust to this new lifestyle, don't become discouraged if you make mistakes. Very few embarking on keto have it all figured out from the start. You may accidentally buy a forbidden fruit or face a cereal craving at breakfast time. It takes time to break old habits and routines.

Just get back on track at the next meal or the next shopping trip. Progress is often two steps forward and one step back.

Grocery shopping for keto resembles an obstacle course at first, with landmines at every turn. But the more you learn about reading labels, planning balanced meals, and substituting higher carb items, the easier it becomes. Keep an open and curious mindset. Experiment with new flavors, recipes and ingredients. Many cultures around the world eat low-carb diets based on whole foods. Look to time-tested, regional cuisines for inspiration.

Along the way, pay attention to how your mind and body respond. Do you feel satisfied after meals? Is your energy stable and mood upbeat? Are cravings diminishing? Track any positive changes to stay motivated, and be sure to celebrate successes, like resisting the siren call of the bakery or discovering a new favorite vegetable.

Remember that perfection is not required. If your cart contains 85% keto-friendly items and 15% indulgences, you're still making significant progress. Any steps to reduce reliance on processed carbs and sugars will benefit your metabolic health. Maintain realistic expectations of yourself as you build knowledge, habits and self-discipline. Once again, this is a marathon, not a sprint.

With preparation, education, and self-compassion, the task of grocery shopping for keto becomes easier over time. The initial effort yields generous dividends through better health, reduced inflammation, and weight loss. Meal planning gets more creative and fulfilling. Your kitchen becomes a domain for nourishing, delicious foods, that nourish your body and satisfy your tastes.

The ketogenic diet connects us to time-honored food traditions focused on whole, minimally processed fare. Shopping the perimeter with mindfulness allows us to opt out of the modern labyrinth of culinary chemicals, additives, and hyper-palatable snack foods. We reclaim agency over our plates.

This chapter provided an overview of strategies for keto success in the grocery aisles. But your journey has only begun. Continue seeking insights and hacks from reputable sources to expand your knowledge.

Experiment, track results, and find staples that work for your lifestyle. Bond with like-minded people for support and ideas.

By taking control of your food environment, you create the optimal conditions for health. Meal by meal, one grocery trip at a time, build the kitchen of your dreams - a space overflowing with ingredients that nourish. Surround yourself with foods that serve your highest good. You'll step into the kitchen each day fueled with inspiration, rather than dread. Grocery shopping becomes an act of self-care.

In closing, be proud of your dedication as you embark on this transformative diet. Trust in the process. Small steps accumulate into massive change over time. The path won't always be easy, but just imagine the vitality and confidence you'll gain. A ketogenic diet pairs beautifully with an active lifestyle, better sleep quality, stress reduction, and other pillars of wellbeing. The journey begins right inside your cart. Shop on with courage and consistency, and savor the bounty of health ahead.

Chapter 6
Mastering Keto Cooking Techniques

In the world of culinary arts, knowing how to cook is just as important as knowing what to cook. This rings particularly true for a keto lifestyle. This chapter is dedicated to helping you master the cooking techniques needed to make the most out of your keto diet.

1. Introduction

The ketogenic diet is high in fats, moderate in proteins, and very low in carbohydrates. This macronutrient composition requires you to rethink your cooking methods. The art of preparing food does not just make meals taste better; it also maximizes the nutritional value, which can be essential in a restrictive diet like keto.

2. Understanding Fats and Oils

One of the first steps in mastering keto cooking is understanding the types of fats and oils you'll be using.

Saturated Fats: These are typically solid at room temperature and are found in foods like butter, lard, and coconut oil. They are stable at high temperatures, making them good for frying and sautéing.

Monounsaturated Fats: These fats are liquid at room temperature and solidify when chilled. Olive oil and avocado oil are high in monounsaturated fats. They are suitable for cooking at medium temperatures.

Polyunsaturated Fats: These fats stay liquid even when refrigerated. They include omega-3 and omega-6 fats, which we get from foods like fatty fish and flaxseeds. They are less stable and should not be used for high-heat cooking.

Knowing which fats to use at what temperatures is key to keto cooking, and using the right fat can elevate the taste and nutrition of your dishes.

3. Sautéing and Stir-frying

Sautéing is a quick, high-heat method of cooking where you rapidly toss food in a small amount of oil in a hot pan. Stir-frying is similar, but usually involves higher heat and constant stirring. Both methods allow you to cook food quickly, which can help preserve nutrients. These methods are excellent for cooking vegetables, seafood, and small or thin pieces of meat.

4. Frying

Deep-frying and pan-frying are techniques that involve cooking food in a lot of oil or fat. While these methods are often associated with unhealthy food, they can be a part of a balanced keto diet when done properly. The key is to choose your oils carefully (opt for saturated and monounsaturated fats) and to keep the temperature under control to avoid burning.

5. Baking and Roasting

Baking and roasting are dry heat cooking methods that are excellent for preparing a wide range of keto-friendly dishes. You can roast meats and vegetables to bring out their flavors. Baking allows you to prepare a wide range of keto bread, cakes, and pastries using low-carb flour alternatives, like almond and coconut flour.

6. Grilling

Grilling imparts a smoky flavor to food that other cooking methods can't replicate. It's an excellent method for cooking meats, fish, and even some vegetables. However, be mindful not to char your food too much, as it can lead to the formation of harmful compounds.

7. Steaming

Steaming is a gentle cooking method that preserves nutrients better than any other. It's excellent for cooking fish, seafood, and non-starchy vegetables. For added flavor, you can steam foods on a bed of herbs or aromatics.

8. Slow Cooking

Using a slow cooker can make keto cooking much more manageable. It's great for cooking large cuts of meat and dense vegetables. All you have to do is add your ingredients and let the slow cooker do its job. Plus, it's perfect for meal prep as it can cook in large quantities.

9. Sous Vide

Sous vide is a method of cooking where food is vacuum-sealed in a bag and then cooked to a precise temperature in a water bath. This technique ensures your meats are perfectly cooked to your desired doneness, and it can bring out flavors you wouldn't achieve with other methods.

10. Poaching

Poaching is a gentle way of cooking that involves submerging food in a liquid just below boiling point. It's an excellent method for cooking delicate foods like eggs, fish, and chicken. While not as common in the keto kitchen, it's a method worth exploring.

11. Braising

Braising involves two steps: searing the food at a high temperature and then finishing it in a covered pot at a lower temperature surrounded by a small amount of liquid. This slow, low-heat method of cooking is perfect for transforming tougher cuts of meat into tender, flavorful dishes.

12. Marinating

Marinating is a technique used to infuse your foods with flavor. It involves soaking your food in a mixture of seasonings, oil, and acid (like vinegar or lemon juice) before cooking. Marinating not only adds flavor but also tenderizes your food, making it more enjoyable to eat. Be sure to use keto-friendly marinades.

13. Seasoning Your Foods

When it comes to flavor, seasoning is key. Beyond salt and pepper, you have a whole array of herbs, spices, and other seasonings to play with. Use these to add variety and interest to your keto dishes. As you gain confidence, don't be afraid to experiment with new flavor combinations.

14. Emulsifying

An emulsion is a mixture of two liquids that don't typically mix well, like oil and water. In a keto kitchen, this comes in handy when making dressings, mayonnaise, and certain sauces. The key to a good emulsion is adding the oil slowly and whisking continuously.

15. Thickening Sauces and Gravies

Traditional thickeners like flour and cornstarch are not keto-friendly. Instead, use alternatives like xanthan gum, glucomannan, or even egg yolks. Remember, a little goes a long way with these thickeners.

16. Dessert Techniques

Desserts on keto are entirely possible, and learning a few essential techniques will help you master this delicious area. Whipping cream into soft peaks, melting chocolate over a bain-marie, and making a meringue are just some of the skills you'll want to develop.

17. Adapting Recipes

One of the most useful skills in a keto kitchen is learning to adapt non-keto recipes. With a bit of creativity, many of your favorite dishes can be transformed into a keto-friendly version.

18. Meal Prepping

Meal prepping is a practice that can make your keto lifestyle much more manageable. Spend a few hours each week preparing your meals in advance, and you'll always have a keto-friendly meal ready when you need it.

19. Making Keto-Friendly Bread

Many people miss the satisfaction of biting into a slice of bread when they switch to keto. Fortunately, you can make your own keto-friendly bread using almond flour, coconut flour, or ground flaxseeds. Learning to bake your own bread can open up a world of keto-friendly sandwiches, toast, and even breadcrumbs for other dishes.

20. Fermenting and Pickling

Fermentation and pickling are age-old methods of preserving food that can be incorporated into a ketogenic diet. Fermented foods like sauerkraut and kimchi are excellent sources of probiotics. Homemade pickles, made without sugar, can add a tart and crunchy element to your meals.

21. Dehydrating

If you own a dehydrator, you can make your own keto-friendly snacks like jerky or vegetable crisps. Dehydrating food is a great way to preserve it while concentrating its flavors.

22. Making Bone Broth

Bone broth is rich in minerals and collagen, making it a nutritious addition to your keto diet. Making bone broth involves simmering animal bones and connective tissue for several hours. This long, slow cooking process allows you to extract as much goodness from the bones as possible.

23. Mastering Omelettes and Scrambled Eggs

Eggs are a staple on the keto diet. Learning to make a good omelette or scrambled eggs is a valuable skill. Remember to cook your eggs gently over low heat to keep them tender.

24. Keto Sushi Rolls

You don't have to give up sushi on a keto diet. Instead of rice, use riced cauliflower to make your sushi rolls. It's a fun and delicious way to enjoy sushi without the carbs.

25. Smoothies and Shakes

Smoothies and shakes can be a quick and easy meal or snack on a ketogenic diet. Using a blender, you can mix protein powder, almond milk or coconut milk, and keto-friendly fruits, like berries or avocado, to make a tasty and filling smoothie.

26. Making Keto Ice Cream

Just because you're on a keto diet doesn't mean you can't enjoy ice cream. By learning to make your own keto-friendly ice cream using heavy cream, almond milk, and a sugar substitute like erythritol, you can satisfy your sweet tooth without the guilt.

27. Infusing Oils and Vinegars

Infusing oils and vinegars with herbs, spices, or garlic, adds an extra dimension of flavor to your keto dishes. They can be used in dressings, marinades, or as a finishing touch to your dishes.

28. Cooking with Keto Flours

Keto baking is an art of its own, and understanding how to work with low-carb flours like almond flour, coconut flour, or flax meal is essential. Each has its own unique properties and is better suited to certain types of recipes.

29. Repurposing Leftovers

A key to success on the keto diet is to always have ready-to-eat, keto-friendly food on hand. One way to do this is by repurposing your leftovers. Turn last night's roasted chicken into a chicken salad for lunch, or use leftover vegetables to make a frittata.

Conclusion

With these cooking techniques under your belt, you're well on your way to becoming a keto kitchen master. Remember, cooking is as much an art as it is a science. There's always something new to learn, a new dish to try, or a new technique to master. So keep exploring, experimenting, and most importantly, enjoying your keto cooking adventure.

Chapter 7
Delicious, Easy-to-Follow Keto Recipes

Embarking on your ketogenic journey doesn't mean you have to give up on the joy of eating. Instead, it provides a new opportunity to get creative and explore new culinary horizons. With a slight adjustment to your shopping list, and a splash of creativity in the kitchen, you can create a host of keto-friendly meals that are both delicious and nourishing. In this chapter, we will take you through some easy-to-follow keto recipes that you can incorporate into your diet.

1. Introduction

The key to enjoying a diverse range of meals on a ketogenic diet is learning how to substitute high-carb ingredients with low-carb alternatives. Fortunately, there are a plethora of options available that can help you recreate your favorite dishes in a keto-friendly way. Let's start by exploring some basic recipes that you can easily make at home.

2. Keto Breakfast Recipes

Breakfast is a crucial meal that sets the tone for your day. Starting with a satisfying and nutrient-rich keto meal can provide you with the energy you need to conquer the day ahead.

2.1. Fluffy Keto Pancakes

Who said pancakes are off the menu on keto? These fluffy, satisfying pancakes are made with almond flour and cream cheese, providing a protein-packed, low-carb start to your day.

Ingredients:

1 cup almond flour
2 large eggs
2 oz cream cheese, softened
1 tsp vanilla extract
1/2 tsp baking powder
1/4 cup unsweetened almond milk
1 tbsp granulated erythritol (or sweetener of choice)
Butter or coconut oil for frying

Instructions:

In a blender, combine all the ingredients until smooth.
Heat a large non-stick skillet over medium heat and grease it lightly with butter or coconut oil.
Pour a 1/4 cup of the batter onto the skillet and cook until bubbles form on the surface of the pancake.
Flip and cook the other side for another minute or until golden brown.
Repeat with the remaining batter.
Serve hot with butter and sugar-free syrup if desired.

2.2. Keto Scrambled Eggs with Avocado

Eggs are an excellent source of protein and healthy fats, making them a staple in the ketogenic diet. This recipe combines the creaminess of scrambled eggs with the richness of avocado for a satisfying, nutrient-dense breakfast.

Ingredients:

4 large eggs
1 ripe avocado
2 tbsp heavy cream
Salt and pepper to taste
1 tbsp butter

Instructions:

Crack the eggs into a bowl and whisk them together with the heavy cream, salt, and pepper.

Heat the butter in a non-stick skillet over medium heat.
Pour in the egg mixture and stir gently until the eggs are softly set.
While the eggs are cooking, slice the avocado.
Serve the scrambled eggs with the sliced avocado on the side.

2.3. Keto Chia Seed Pudding

Chia seeds are full of fiber and omega-3 fatty acids, making them a fantastic addition to your keto diet. This pudding can be prepped the night before for a quick, on-the-go breakfast.

Ingredients:

1/4 cup chia seeds
1 cup unsweetened almond milk
1/2 tsp vanilla extract
1 tbsp granulated erythritol (or sweetener of choice)
A pinch of salt
Fresh berries (optional)

Instructions:

In a bowl, mix the chia seeds, almond milk, vanilla extract, sweetener, and salt.
Cover the bowl and place it in the refrigerator overnight.
In the morning, give the pudding a good stir to break up any clumps.
Serve chilled with fresh berries on top, if desired.

3. Keto Lunch and Dinner Recipes

Maintaining variety in your meals is crucial to sustaining a healthy, balanced diet. Here are some keto-friendly lunch and dinner recipes that you can easily prepare at home.

3.1. Keto Chicken Caesar Salad

This classic Caesar salad is keto-friendly, filled with crunchy romaine lettuce, tender chicken, and creamy dressing. It's a delicious, light meal that will keep you satisfied.

Sophia Ramos

Ingredients:

For the salad:

2 chicken breasts, cooked and sliced
1 head of romaine lettuce, chopped
1/4 cup Parmesan cheese, grated
For the dressing:

1/2 cup mayonnaise
1/4 cup Parmesan cheese, grated
2 tbsp lemon juice
1 garlic clove, minced
Salt and pepper to taste

Instructions:

In a large bowl, combine the chopped lettuce, sliced chicken, and Parmesan cheese.
In a separate bowl, whisk together the mayonnaise, Parmesan cheese, lemon juice, garlic, salt, and pepper.
Drizzle the dressing over the salad and toss until well combined.
Serve immediately.

3.2. Keto Zucchini Noodles with Pesto

Zucchini noodles (also known as zoodles) are a fantastic low-carb alternative to pasta. Paired with a flavorful pesto sauce, this dish is both satisfying and refreshing.

Ingredients:

2 large zucchinis
1/2 cup pesto sauce
Salt and pepper to taste
Parmesan cheese, for serving

Instructions:

Use a spiralizer to turn the zucchinis into noodles.

Heat a large pan over medium heat and add the zucchini noodles.

Sauté the noodles for 2-3 minutes until they're heated through. Be careful not to overcook them, or they will become mushy.

Stir in the pesto sauce and toss until the noodles are well coated.

Season with salt and pepper.

Serve hot with a sprinkle of Parmesan cheese on top.

3.3. Keto Bacon-Wrapped Asparagus

Bacon-wrapped asparagus is a delicious and easy-to-make side dish that's perfect for any meal. It's a wonderful way to enjoy your veggies while getting in some extra protein and fats.

Ingredients:

16 asparagus spears
8 slices of bacon
Salt and pepper to taste

Instructions:

Preheat your oven to 400°F (200°C).

Wrap each pair of asparagus spears with a slice of bacon.

Place the wrapped spears on a baking sheet and season with salt and pepper.

Bake for 15-20 minutes, or until the bacon is crispy and the asparagus is tender.

Serve warm.

4. Keto Snack Recipes

Snacks can be a great way to curb hunger between meals and make sure you're getting enough calories and nutrients. Here are some simple, delicious keto snacks you can prepare at home.

4.1. Keto Guacamole

Guacamole is a healthy, delicious snack that's perfect for the keto diet. Rich in healthy fats from avocados, it's perfect for dipping celery sticks, cucumber slices, or keto-friendly chips.

Ingredients:

2 ripe avocados
1/2 red onion, finely chopped
1 small tomato, finely chopped
1 jalapeño pepper, seeds removed and finely chopped (optional)
2 tbsp fresh cilantro, finely chopped
Juice of 1 lime
Salt to taste

Instructions:

Cut the avocados in half, remove the pits, and scoop the flesh into a bowl.

Mash the avocado flesh with a fork until it reaches your desired consistency.

Add the red onion, tomato, jalapeño (if using), cilantro, lime juice, and salt. Mix until well combined.

Taste and adjust the seasoning if needed.

Serve immediately or cover with plastic wrap and refrigerate until ready to serve.

4.2. Keto Cheese Crackers

These keto cheese crackers are made with almond flour and cheese, making them a satisfying low-carb snack.

Ingredients:

1 cup almond flour
1 cup sharp cheddar cheese, grated
1/2 tsp garlic powder
1/4 tsp salt
1 large egg

Instructions:

Preheat your oven to 350°F (175°C) and line a baking sheet with parchment paper.

In a bowl, combine the almond flour, cheese, garlic powder, and salt.

Beat the egg in a separate bowl, then add it to the dry ingredients. Mix until a dough forms.

Place the dough on the prepared baking sheet and roll it out as thin as you can.

Cut the dough into squares with a pizza cutter or knife.

Bake for 12-15 minutes, or until the crackers are golden brown.

Allow the crackers to cool on the baking sheet before serving.

5. Keto Dessert Recipes

Even on a keto diet, there's always room for dessert! These sweet treats are low in carbs and high in flavor.

5.1. Keto Chocolate Mousse

This keto chocolate mousse is a heavenly, creamy dessert that will satisfy your sweet tooth without breaking your carb count.

Ingredients:

1 cup heavy cream
1/2 cup unsweetened cocoa powder
2 tbsp granulated erythritol (or sweetener of choice)
1/2 tsp vanilla extract

Instructions:

Whip the heavy cream in a large bowl until it forms soft peaks.

In a separate bowl, combine the cocoa powder, sweetener, and vanilla extract.

Gradually fold the cocoa mixture into the whipped cream until well combined.

Spoon the mousse into serving dishes and refrigerate for at least 1 hour before serving.

5.2. Keto Almond Flour Cookies

These almond flour cookies are a delicious treat that's low in carbs and easy to make. You can add different flavors, such as cinnamon or cocoa, to vary the taste.

Ingredients:

2 cups almond flour
1/2 cup
1/2 cup granulated erythritol (or sweetener of choice)
1/2 tsp baking powder
1/2 cup unsalted butter, melted
1 tsp vanilla extract

Instructions:

Preheat your oven to 350°F (175°C) and line a baking sheet with parchment paper.
In a bowl, combine the almond flour, sweetener, and baking powder.
Add the melted butter and vanilla extract to the dry ingredients. Mix until a dough forms.
Scoop out tablespoons of dough and roll them into balls. Place the balls on the prepared baking sheet and flatten them with the bottom of a glass.
Bake for 10-12 minutes, or until the edges are golden brown.
Allow the cookies to cool on the baking sheet before serving.

5.3. Keto Cheesecake

This keto cheesecake is creamy and rich, with a sweet almond flour crust and a velvety cream cheese filling. It's a perfect treat for special occasions or just when you need something a little indulgent.

Ingredients:

For the crust:

2 cups almond flour
1/2 cup unsalted butter, melted
2 tbsp granulated erythritol (or sweetener of choice)
For the filling:

4 cups cream cheese, softened
1 cup granulated erythritol (or sweetener of choice)
3 large eggs
1 tsp vanilla extract
Zest of 1 lemon

Instructions:

Preheat your oven to 325°F (163°C) and grease a 9-inch (23 cm) springform pan.

Combine the almond flour, melted butter, and sweetener in a bowl to make the crust. Press the mixture into the bottom of the prepared pan.

Bake the crust for 10 minutes, then remove it from the oven and set it aside.

In a large bowl, beat the cream cheese and sweetener until smooth. Add the eggs one at a time, beating well after each addition. Stir in the vanilla extract and lemon zest.

Pour the cream cheese mixture over the crust in the pan.

Bake for 50-60 minutes, or until the center is set and the top is lightly browned.

Allow the cheesecake to cool in the pan on a wire rack for 10 minutes, then run a knife around the edge of the pan to loosen the cheesecake.

Cool the cheesecake in the pan for 1 hour, then refrigerate it for at least 4 hours before serving.

Conclusion

Creating delicious, satisfying meals on a keto diet doesn't have to be complicated. With these easy-to-follow recipes, you can enjoy a variety of dishes that are high in fat, moderate in protein, and low in carbs. Whether you're new to the ketogenic diet or a seasoned veteran, these recipes are sure to become favorites in your keto meal rotation. And remember, the key to successful dieting is to enjoy what you're eating. Bon appétit!

Chapter 8
Overcoming Common Keto Challenges

Making the switch to a ketogenic diet can require significant changes for many people. Transitioning your body's primary fuel source from carbohydrates to fat and entering a state of ketosis doesn't happen instantly. It takes commitment, preparation, and adaptability to overcome the hurdles that may arise. This chapter provides comprehensive guidance on handling the most common challenges individuals face when adopting a keto lifestyle. We will explore the underlying reasons these issues occur, as well as solutions and tips to power through them smoothly. With knowledge and perseverance, these obstacles can be managed for successful keto adaptation.

One of the most frequently reported challenges upon starting keto is commonly referred to as the "keto flu." This refers to flu-like symptoms that may arise during the first one to two weeks as your body transitions into ketosis. Common keto flu symptoms include headaches, fatigue and low energy, nausea, dizziness and foggy thinking, difficulty sleeping, irritability, cramps, and constipation. These symptoms arise because your body is accustomed to using glucose from carbohydrates for fuel. As carb intake is drastically reduced, your body needs time to learn to produce and utilize ketones from fat for energy instead. This transition period can temporarily disrupt energy levels, electrolyte balance, hydration, and other bodily functions, provoking the keto flu. Fortunately, the keto flu is usually temporary, lasting about one to three weeks as your body adapts. Still, symptoms can impact daily life, so it's worth utilizing strategies to minimize their severity.

Here are some tips: Stay hydrated by drinking plenty of water and mineral-rich broths, as hydration is key for flushing out the metabolic byproducts causing symptoms. Manage electrolytes by consuming bone broth, leafy greens, avocados, and pink salt to replenish sodium, magnesium, and potassium. Consider taking a supplement too. Eat enough calories and don't restrict when adapting to keto, as consuming adequate fat and protein helps ease the transition. Get enough rest by allowing your body time to adapt by getting 7-9 hours of sleep nightly, as rest supports the transition. Exercise lightly with activities like walking or yoga, but avoid intense workouts that may prolong the keto flu. Wait it out and accept that the keto flu is temporary - within a few weeks, as your body adapts, symptoms will subside. With proper hydration, electrolyte replenishment, mild activity, and ample rest, the keto flu can be managed. Take it easy on yourself mentally and physically to adapt more smoothly. The discomfort is temporary and worth it for the long-term benefits.

Constipation is another common complaint, especially in the first few weeks of ketosis. Reduced fiber and hydration along with dietary changes impact bowel regularity. Luckily, proactive steps can lessen constipation: Drink plenty of fluids daily, aiming for 2-4 liters of total fluids, as proper hydration keeps bowels functioning well. Include natural fiber sources like leafy greens, chia, flax, and non-starchy veggies which add fiber that promotes regularity. Add magnesium-rich foods like spinach, avocado, almonds and dark chocolate which relax the bowels. Exercise regularly, as physical movement stimulates the bowels and digestive tract. Consider probiotic foods like sauerkraut, kimchi, kefir, and yogurt which contain probiotics that support healthy digestion. Use care with constipating foods like dairy, eggs, and low-fiber products, which can be constipating, so enjoy in moderation. Try herbal teas with anti-inflammatory properties that can aid digestion, like peppermint, ginger and chamomile.

Additionally, be patient. It takes some time for your gastrointestinal system to adapt to dietary changes. Consistency is key. The potential for constipation and other mild digestive troubles should subside within a few weeks as your body adjusts. Don't hesitate to consult a healthcare professional if severe issues persist.

Feeling drained, both mentally and physically, is not uncommon, especially in the initial few weeks of transitioning to keto. Your body is accustomed to utilizing glucose for quick energy. As glucose becomes scarcer, and your body adapts to creating ketones for fuel, fatigue is a typical side effect. Remember, this is temporary. Here are some tips for overcoming low energy and weakness: Be sure you're eating enough calories and fat, as this gives your body the fuel it needs. Too significant of a deficit can backfire and cause fatigue. Replenish electrolytes, like sodium, magnesium, and potassium which are essential for energy levels. Stay hydrated, as dehydration exacerbates fatigue - drink plenty of water throughout the day. Watch caffeine intake.While a moderate amount of coffee is fine for an energy boost, excess caffeine can disrupt sleep and hydration, compounding fatigue. Get plenty of rest by allowing your body time to adapt by getting 7-9 hours of quality sleep per night. Exercise moderately with light walking and gentle yoga which help, but avoid intense workouts that may prolong fatigue until adapted. Go easier initially when energy is lower. Avoid overexerting yourself physically until adapted, by pacing yourself and not pushing too hard until your body adjusts.

Be patient with yourself. Listen to your body. Nurture it with ample rest, minerals, hydration, and nutrition during this transition. The period of lower energy, lethargy, and weakness will pass, as you become keto adapted.

Cravings for sweets, bread, pasta, and other high-carb favorites are very common in the early stages of keto adaptation. Your body is used to regular spikes of glucose from these foods and will send signals requesting more to maintain homeostasis. But rest assured, these intense cravings are temporary. As you become adapted to fat-burning, they will fade. Here are some tips for combating sugar and carb cravings in the meantime: Eat regularly by not skipping meals which leads to cravings, so stay satisfied by eating every 4-6 hours. Manage stress, as emotional or chronic stress amplifies cravings, so adopt stress-reduction practices like meditation, yoga, or brisk walking to help. Get quality sleep, as lack of sleep disrupts hormone signals, so aim for 7-9 hours nightly. Stay hydrated and replenish electrolytes, as thirst signals can seem like food cravings, so drink sufficient water and get minerals. Increase healthy fats to help stabilize blood sugar and manage cravings. Choose keto-friendly sweets like small portions of low-carb treats made with stevia or monk fruit. Find distraction by shifting your focus to an enjoyable activity whenever an intense craving strikes. Be patient, and remind yourself that cravings will diminish over time, as your body adapts to fat-burning.

Consistency and commitment are vital in the initial phases of keto adaptation. The intensity of sugar and carb cravings should lessen around the 3-4 week mark, as your body learns to utilize ketones efficiently, for fuel.

Sleep disturbances like insomnia are not uncommon when first transitioning to a keto diet. This results from multiple factors including low carb intake, altered hormone function, electrolyte imbalance, and sometimes too much dietary fat eaten close to bedtime. But there are solutions for managing keto-related sleep troubles: Avoid screens before bedtime, as blue light from electronics inhibits melatonin production, so unwind tech-free 30-60 minutes before bed. Establish a calming pre-bed routine like light yoga, reading, or meditation to help prepare the body for restful sleep. Keep your sleep environment dark, cool, and comfortable by blocking out light and reducing noise or other distractions. Be consistent with sleep and wake times by maintaining a regular schedule to support your circadian rhythm. Avoid caffeine after 2 pm since caffeine's effects last many hours, disrupting sleep. Limit carbs to 1-2 g net carbs in your evening meal or snack to prevent blood sugar spikes that can disrupt sleep. Supplement magnesium before bed as it promotes muscle relaxation and sleepiness. Use sleep aids like melatonin, magnesium, or over-the-counter sleep aids as needed to provide temporary help getting to sleep. Exercise regularly, but not before bed, as movement helps sleep, but vigorous evening exercise may hinder it. Be patient as it can take 3-4 weeks for sleep to normalize as your body gets keto adapted.

With consistency and time, your sleep is likely to regulate as your body adapts to utilizing fat and ketones for fuel. Don't hesitate to consult your healthcare provider if insomnia or sleep troubles persist.

Because insulin levels and carb intake drop sharply on keto, the kidneys excrete more sodium and fluids than normal in the adaptation phase. This makes dehydration and electrolyte imbalance a common side effect initially. Symptoms may include fatigue and lethargy, muscle cramping, headaches, dizziness, constipation, increased thirst, and heart palpitations. Luckily this can be easily managed with proper hydration and electrolyte replenishment: Drink ample fluids aiming for 2-4 liters of total fluids daily, choosing water, herbal tea, and bone broth. Focus on getting sufficient sodium, magnesium and potassium from foods like avocados, nuts, leafy greens, salmon, and bone broth. Using a mineral salt provides sodium and trace minerals. Consider a daily electrolyte supplement to ensure adequate replenishment as your body adapts. Eat foods rich in magnesium like dark leafy greens, nuts, seeds, and dark chocolate which supports nerve and muscle function. Increase potassium via avocado, mushrooms, salmon, and beef, which helps regulate hydration and blood pressure.

With consistent hydration and daily electrolyte replenishment from natural food sources and supplements, symptoms should subside within a few weeks as your body adapts to the keto diet.

From constipation, to diarrhea and bloating, some mild GI distress can arise when transitioning to keto. Your digestive system is adjusting to different macronutrients, reduced fiber, and fewer gut-friendly carbs. This disruption can provoke issues like constipation, diarrhea, gas and bloating, heartburn, and stomach cramping. The good news is that these issues usually resolve within a few weeks as your gut microbiome adapts. Be proactive with the following: Eat plenty of low-carb vegetables for fiber, which helps move food through the GI tract. Stay hydrated with 2-3 liters of fluids daily to prevent constipation, by drinking water and mineral-rich bone broth. Incorporate prebiotic and probiotic foods, like sauerkraut, kimchi, kefir and yogurt, which help nurture gut microbes. Eating high-quality fats, such as coconut, olive, and avocado oils support gut health. Reduce dairy and nuts if bloating occurs to limit hard-to-digest foods. Avoid sugar alcohols initially as sorbitol and xylitol supplements can provoke bloating and gas. Manage stress levels since stress exacerbates GI issues, so adopt soothing practices like yoga, deep breathing, and meditation.

With patience and consistency, your gut should adapt within several weeks, resulting in more comfortable digestion. Avoid eliminating too many plant foods or fiber to prevent exacerbating GI troubles.

Making the switch to being fueled primarily by fat instead of carbs, takes some getting used to. Some find it challenging at first to eat enough fat to meet the high-fat goals of keto without going overboard on protein and calories. Here are tips for getting enough healthy fats in your keto diet: Cook with fatty cuts of meat and bone-in poultry which provide a hefty dose of fat. Choose high-fat dairy like cheese, heavy cream and full-fat sour cream, but be mindful of dairy tolerance. Snack on nuts, seeds and their butters which are very high in healthy fats. Eat avocados and olives often as they're a tasty way to add monounsaturated fats. Incorporate oils like olive, avocado, and coconut into cooking and dressings. Add butter or ghee into sauces, vegetables, and grain-free baked goods. Mix in high-fat ingredients like heavy cream, cream cheese, pesto, or coconut butter into recipes. Choose fattier cuts of fish like salmon, or try fish oil supplements. Drink bulletproof coffee made with butter, MCT, or coconut oil for a quick fat boost.

With planning and creativity, getting adequate fat each day is very doable. Dietary fat enhances flavor and satisfaction, helping you feel fuller and more content with your keto diet over time.

When transitioning to keto, overdoing it on dietary fats can provoke some unpleasant symptoms. Many make the mistake of going overboard on fat intake, especially saturated fat, when starting keto. Issues like nausea, diarrhea, and acid reflux may occur. To avoid these unpleasant symptoms, tailor fat intake to your personal tolerance: Gradually increase fat intake, not all at once, allowing your body, gallbladder and digestion to adapt. Limit portions of very high-fat foods if they cause distress, as smaller portions may be better tolerated. Choose fattier cuts of meat and poultry rather than organ meats, skin or suet, if these trigger issues. Limit added fats like coconut oil and butter if these aggravate discomfort - stick to naturally fatty foods instead. Avoid going extremely high in fat, especially saturated fat, all at once by increasing fat intake slowly. Ensure adequate hydration and electrolytes to support fat digestion. Back down your fat intake if symptoms arise and increase slowly, as your body needs time to adapt to higher fat intake.

Patience and moderation are key to preventing adverse reactions when transitioning to a higher fat intake. Target the minimum level of fat needed to maintain ketosis and satiety as your body adjusts.

In ketosis, trace amounts of acetone, a ketone body, are exhaled causing "keto breath." This rotten fruit-like smell is a harmless side effect of fat breakdown. But it can be unpleasant. Here are some tips to lessen keto breath: Drink more water to help dilute acetone levels by staying hydrated. Use mouthwash and brush regularly to maintain excellent oral hygiene. Chew mint gum or use lozenges as peppermint helps mask odors temporarily. Increase greens and cruciferous veggies which help balance pH levels linked to odor. Avoid severely restricting carbs for extended periods, as occasional carb cycling helps rebalance pH. Consider activated charcoal or chlorophyll supplements as some find these help reduce odor.

For most, keto breath diminishes in the adaptation phase as the body becomes efficient at fat burning. If it persists, investigate potential underlying causes like infection or metabolic changes. But typically, the smell is just an inconvenience that lessens over time.

Along with keto breath, a temporary metallic, chemical, or unpleasant taste in the mouth can occur. Like the breath odor, this stems from ketone production and accompanies the transition into ketosis. Here are some suggestions to combat a persistent unpleasant taste: Drink more water and stay hydrated, as this helps dilute ketones. Use antibacterial mouthwash to eliminate bacteria that may impact taste. Brush your tongue when brushing teeth to scrape away buildup contributing to taste. Chew mint gum or have mints on hand as minty flavors help mask unpleasant taste temporarily. Rinse your mouth with lemon water as citrus helps neutralize odors. Wait it out, as for most, this resolves fully within 4-6 weeks as the body adapts to ketosis.

Thankfully, this unwanted taste is just temporary for most individuals as their body adapts to ketone production and utilization. If it persists long-term or is severe, consult your healthcare provider to check for underlying illness. But typically, the taste is just an inconvenience that lessens over time.

Some individuals may experience occasional heart palpitations and irregular heart rhythms when transitioning into ketosis. While alarming, this is typically harmless in an otherwise healthy person. Potential reasons include electrolyte imbalances as levels adjust, especially magnesium, potassium and sodium, so supplement if needed. Dehydration and increased excretion of minerals can also provoke heart flutters, so drink plenty of mineral-rich fluids. Adrenalin release triggered by lower glucose levels and metabolic changes may be a factor, but this subsides as the body adapts. Too drastic a calorie deficit stresses the body, so eat an appropriate amount of calories. Caffeine sensitivity may be heightened by keto, so limit or avoid caffeine if palpitations occur. Nicotine can also exacerbate palpitations, so avoid smoking while adapting to keto. While unsettling, heart palpitations while adapting to keto are usually not harmful. However, consult your doctor to rule out underlying conditions, and immediately seek help if palpitations are prolonged, severe or accompanied by chest pain.

Chapter 9

Keto and Exercise: A Comprehensive Guide

Exercise is a crucial component of a healthy lifestyle, regardless of the diet you follow. When combined with the ketogenic diet, regular physical activity can help accelerate weight loss, improve body composition, and enhance overall health and well-being. However, when adopting a ketogenic diet, understanding the way your body uses energy during exercise, is key to maximizing your workouts. This chapter will guide you through the intricate relationship between a keto diet and exercise.

1. Understanding Energy Metabolism During Exercise

When you exercise, your body needs energy. This energy comes from either glucose, derived from carbohydrates, or fats. The source your body uses depends on the intensity and duration of the exercise.

In a non-keto-adapted state, your body uses glucose as its primary fuel source during high-intensity exercises, such as sprinting or weight lifting. For low to moderate-intensity exercises like jogging or cycling at a relaxed pace, your body uses a mix of glucose and fats. When you're keto-adapted, however, your body switches to using fats as its primary energy source.

2. The Shift to Ketogenic Metabolism

When you start a ketogenic diet, your body goes through a transition period as it shifts from burning glucose to burning fat for energy. This is called becoming "keto-adapted." During this transition, you might experience a temporary decrease in energy and athletic performance. However, once your body becomes adapted to using fat for fuel, your energy levels should return to normal or even increase.

3. The Impact of Keto on Endurance Performance

Several studies suggest that a ketogenic diet can benefit endurance athletes. Once keto-adapted, athletes have a virtually unlimited supply of calories from stored body fat to fuel their performance. This can be a significant advantage in endurance events, as athletes can avoid "hitting the wall" —which is a state of exhaustion that can occur when the body's stored glucose, or glycogen, runs out.

4. The Impact of Keto on High-Intensity Performance

The research on the impact of a ketogenic diet on high-intensity performance is mixed. Some studies suggest a possible decrease in performance, while others show no change. This is because high-intensity activities typically rely on glucose for energy, which is limited on a keto diet.

However, after an adaptation period, many athletes can perform high-intensity activities while in ketosis by utilizing ketones and the small amount of glucose produced by the liver. The key is to allow your body sufficient time to adapt to the diet before evaluating its impact on your high-intensity performance.

5. The Impact of Keto on Muscle Mass

There's a common misconception that it's difficult to maintain or gain muscle mass on a ketogenic diet due to the low intake of carbohydrates. However, research has shown that a well-formulated ketogenic diet can support muscle maintenance and growth. Adequate protein intake and resistance training are key in preserving muscle mass while on a keto diet.

6. Hydration and Electrolytes

Hydration and electrolyte balance are crucial when exercising, especially on a ketogenic diet. When you're in ketosis, your body tends to excrete more water and electrolytes. This, combined with the fluid loss that occurs during exercise, can quickly lead to dehydration if not properly managed.

Make sure you're drinking plenty of water before, during, and after your workout. Also, replenish electrolytes, particularly sodium, potassium, and magnesium, by consuming electrolyte-rich foods or supplements.

7. Fueling Your Workouts on Keto

Planning your meals around your workouts can optimize energy levels and performance. While timing isn't everything, eating your largest meal after your workout can help replenish energy stores and support muscle repair and growth. Eating a balanced meal with adequate protein, healthy fats, and low-carb vegetables can also help you recover from your workouts more effectively.

If you exercise first thing in the morning, and prefer to do so in a fasted state, it's still important to replenish your body afterward. A protein-rich breakfast can kick start muscle repair and growth, and adding healthy fats can provide a sustained energy source for the rest of the day.

8. Pre and Post-Workout Snacks

Pre-workout snacks on a keto diet should aim to provide a slow and steady source of energy. Foods high in healthy fats, moderate in protein, and low in carbs are ideal. Some options include avocados, nuts, seeds, and protein shakes made with unsweetened almond milk or full-fat Greek yogurt.

Post-workout snacks should help restore muscle glycogen, repair muscle damage, and promote muscle growth. Consider consuming a combination of protein for muscle recovery and healthy fats for satiety. A protein shake, eggs with avocado, or a chicken salad with olive oil are excellent choices.

9. Supplements for Exercise on a Keto Diet

Certain supplements can enhance your exercise performance and recovery while on a ketogenic diet.

MCT Oil: Medium-chain triglyceride (MCT) oil can be converted quickly into ketones, providing a rapid energy source during your workouts.

Creatine: This supplement can increase strength and muscle mass, and it may be especially beneficial for high-intensity workouts.

Beta-Alanine: Beta-Alanine can help buffer acid in muscles, improving performance during high-intensity and short-duration exercises.

Branched-Chain Amino Acids (BCAAs): BCAAs can help promote muscle recovery and reduce exercise-induced muscle soreness.

Electrolyte Supplements: These can help maintain hydration and electrolyte balance during longer or more intense workouts.

Remember, supplements should not replace a balanced diet, complement it. Always consult a healthcare professional before adding any new supplements to your regimen.

10. Recovery After Exercise

Recovery is just as important as the exercise itself. Giving your body time to rest and repair can improve your performance and gains over time. A combination of adequate sleep, proper nutrition, hydration, and stretching or mobility exercises, can support optimal recovery.

11. Balancing Macronutrients for Exercise

When engaging in regular exercise on a ketogenic diet, it's important to strike a balance between your macronutrients which arefats, proteins, and carbohydrates. While carbohydrates are typically limited on a keto diet, they still play a role in providing energy for intense workouts.

How to Balance Macronutrients for Exercise

For low to moderate-intensity workouts, sticking to a standard ketogenic diet with moderate protein intake and minimal carbs should suffice. However, for high-intensity or prolonged endurance exercises, some individuals may benefit from a targeted ketogenic diet (TKD) or cyclical ketogenic diet (CKD).

TKD involves consuming a small amount of easily digestible carbohydrates before and/or after workouts to provide an additional energy source. This can help support intense exercise performance without disrupting ketosis.

CKD involves cycling between periods of strict keto eating and higher carbohydrate intake. Typically, this involves a few days of strict keto followed by a "carb-loading" period before intense workouts. This approach can be beneficial for those engaging in highly demanding physical activities.

It's important to note that the TKD and CKD approaches are more advanced and may not be suitable or necessary for everyone. If you're unsure, consulting with a healthcare professional or registered dietitian who specializes in ketogenic diets can provide personalized guidance.

12. Listening to Your Body

Every individual is unique, and what works for one person may not work for another. It's crucial to listen to your body and make adjustments as needed.

How to Listen to Your Body

Pay attention to how you feel during and after workouts. If you notice a decrease in energy, performance, or recovery, it may be an indication that you need to adjust your macronutrient intake, timing of meals, or overall calorie intake. Experiment with different approaches and find what works best for you.

Additionally, be mindful of any signs of overtraining or burnout. Pushing yourself too hard without proper rest and recovery can have negative consequences on your health and progress. Allow yourself adequate rest days and prioritize quality sleep.

13. Modifying Your Exercise Routine

As you transition to a ketogenic diet, you may find that your exercise performance and endurance fluctuate. It's normal to experience some adjustments and modifications to your routine.

How to Modify Your Exercise Routine

Consider reducing the intensity or duration of your workouts during the initial stages of keto adaptation. Focus on maintaining consistency and gradually increasing the intensity as your body becomes more accustomed to using fat for fuel.

Incorporating different types of exercises, such as strength training, cardiovascular activities, and flexibility exercises, can help maintain a well-rounded fitness routine. Experiment with different activities to find what you enjoy and what complements your keto lifestyle.

14. Seeking Professional Guidance

If you have specific fitness goals, pre-existing health conditions, or concerns about exercise on a ketogenic diet, it's advisable to seek guidance from professionals who specialize in both nutrition and fitness.

How to Seek Professional Guidance

A registered dietitian or nutritionist can provide personalized recommendations on macronutrient ratios, supplementation, and meal timing based on your individual needs and goals. Additionally, working with a qualified fitness trainer or coach who understands the ketogenic diet can help you design an exercise program that aligns with your dietary preferences and optimizes your results.

15. Mental Benefits of Exercise on Keto

Exercise not only benefits the body but also has numerous mental health benefits. Engaging in physical activity while on a ketogenic diet can contribute to improved mood, reduced stress levels, and increased mental clarity.

How Exercise Benefits Mental Health on Keto

Exercise releases endorphins, the feel-good hormones that boost mood and promote a sense of well-being. Regular exercise has been shown to reduce symptoms of anxiety and depression, enhance cognitive function, and improve sleep quality.

When combined with a ketogenic diet, exercise can further enhance mental clarity and focus, due to the steady supply of ketones to the brain. This can be particularly beneficial for individuals who experience brain fog or mental fatigue.

16. Incorporating Different Types of Exercise

To reap the full benefits of exercise on a ketogenic diet, it's important to incorporate a variety of activities into your routine. This ensures you're working different muscle groups, improving cardiovascular health, and maintaining flexibility.

Types of Exercise to Include

Resistance Training: Engage in strength training exercises, such as lifting weights or using resistance bands, to build and maintain muscle mass. This is especially important on a keto diet to prevent muscle loss.

Cardiovascular Exercise: Incorporate aerobic activities like jogging, cycling, swimming, or brisk walking to improve cardiovascular fitness and burn calories.

Flexibility and Mobility: Include exercises such as yoga, Pilates, or stretching routines, to improve flexibility, joint mobility, and posture.

HIIT (High-Intensity Interval Training): Consider adding HIIT workouts, which involve short bursts of intense activity followed by short recovery periods. HIIT can help improve endurance, increase calorie burn, and boost metabolism.

Outdoor Activities: Take advantage of outdoor activities like hiking, biking, or playing sports to enjoy nature while staying active.

17. Staying Motivated and Setting Goals

Maintaining motivation and setting realistic goals are crucial for long-term success in both your ketogenic diet and exercise routine.

How to Stay Motivated and Set Goals

Set Specific Goals: Define specific and measurable goals that align with your overall health and fitness objectives. These goals can be related to weight loss, strength gains, endurance improvements, or any other fitness parameter that is meaningful to you.

Track Your Progress: Keep a record of your workouts, measurements, and achievements. This will help you track your progress over time and provide motivation to continue.

Find an Accountability Partner: Having a workout buddy or joining a supportive community can provide the motivation and accountability needed to stay consistent with your exercise routine.

Celebrate Milestones: Celebrate your accomplishments along the way, whether it's reaching a weight loss milestone, achieving a new personal record in your workouts, or completing a fitness challenge. Rewarding yourself for your hard work can reinforce positive behaviors.

18. Safety Precautions and Listening to Your Body

When starting a new exercise regimen, it's important to prioritize safety and listen to your body's signals to prevent injury.

Safety Precautions for Exercise on Keto

Warm-Up and Cool-Down: Always include a warm-up and cool-down period in your workouts to prepare your body and prevent injury.

Gradual Progression: Start with manageable intensity and gradually increase the duration and intensity of your workouts over time. Avoid pushing yourself too hard, too quickly.

Pay Attention to Recovery: Allow your body enough time to recover between workouts to prevent overtraining and burnout. Adequate rest is essential for muscle repair and overall performance.

Consult a Healthcare Professional: If you have any underlying health conditions or concerns about engaging in certain types of exercise, consult with a healthcare professional before starting a new exercise program.

Conclusion

Combining a ketogenic diet with regular exercise can lead to significant improvements in physical and mental health. By understanding energy metabolism, balancing macronutrients, listening to your body, and incorporating different types of exercise, you can optimize the benefits of both practices. Stay motivated, set realistic goals, and prioritize safety to ensure long-term success on your keto and exercise journey. Remember, consistency and patience are key, and always consult with professionals for personalized guidance.

Chapter 10

Keto for the Long Haul: Sustainability and Adaptation

Embarking on a ketogenic diet is not just about short-term results; it's about adopting a sustainable lifestyle that supports your health and well-being in the long run. This chapter focuses on strategies for maintaining ketosis, adapting to different situations, and ensuring the sustainability of your keto journey.

1. Finding Your Sustainable Approach

While the ketogenic diet provides a framework for carbohydrate restriction and fat adaptation, there are various approaches within the keto spectrum. It's essential to find the version that works best for you and is sustainable in the long term.

Determining Your Sustainable Approach

Consider factors such as personal preferences, lifestyle, cultural influences, and health goals when determining your sustainable approach to the keto diet. Some individuals may thrive on a strict and precise approach, while others may prefer a more flexible or intuitive approach. Experimentation and self-reflection will help you find the balance that works for you.

2. Adapting to Different Situations

Throughout your keto journey, you will encounter different situations that may challenge your dietary choices. Learning how to adapt and make keto-friendly choices in various settings will help you maintain consistency.

Adapting to Social Events

Navigating social events while on a ketogenic diet can be a challenge. When attending parties or gatherings, communicate your dietary preferences to the host in advance, offer to bring a keto-friendly dish, or focus on the protein and vegetable options available. Being prepared and proactive will help you stick to your dietary choices without feeling deprived.

Traveling on Keto

Traveling, whether for business or pleasure, requires some extra planning to stay on track with your keto diet. Research restaurants and grocery stores at your destination that offer keto-friendly options. Pack keto-friendly snacks, such as nuts or low-carb protein bars, for convenient on-the-go options. If you have access to a kitchen, consider renting accommodations that allow you to prepare your own meals.

Eating Out on Keto

Eating out at restaurants can still be enjoyable and keto-friendly. Look for dishes that contain quality protein sources, healthy fats, and non-starchy vegetables. Be mindful of hidden sugars or high-carb ingredients in sauces or dressings. Don't be afraid to ask for modifications or substitutions to make a dish fit your dietary needs.

3. Flexibility within Keto

While maintaining ketosis is the primary goal of a ketogenic diet, allowing for flexibility within the diet can make it more sustainable in the long term.

Cyclical Ketogenic Diet (CKD)

The CKD involves cycling between periods of strict keto eating and higher carbohydrate intake. This approach can be beneficial for athletes or individuals who engage in intense workouts and require more carbohydrates for optimal performance. It allows for replenishing glycogen stores while still maintaining a predominantly ketogenic lifestyle.

Targeted Ketogenic Diet (TKD)

The TKD involves consuming a small amount of easily digestible carbohydrates before and/or after workouts. This provides an additional energy source for intense physical activity while remaining in ketosis for the majority of the time.

4. Staying Accountable and Tracking Progress

Accountability and tracking progress are essential tools for maintaining motivation and ensuring long-term success on a keto diet.

Using Food Tracking Apps

Food tracking apps, such as MyFitnessPal or Carb Manager, can help you monitor your macronutrient intake, track your progress, and ensure you're staying within your desired keto range. They also provide insights into your nutrient consumption, allowing you to make adjustments if needed.

Keeping a Food Journal

In addition to using food tracking apps, keeping a food journal can help you reflect on your eating patterns, identify triggers for overeating or cravings, and track any changes in your energy levels or well-being. It can serve as a valuable tool for self-awareness and identifying areas for improvement.

Regular Check-Ins and Measurements

Schedule regular check-ins with yourself to evaluate your progress, reassess your goals, and make necessary adjustments. Take measurements of your body, such as weight, body measurements, or body composition, to track changes over time. Remember that progress goes beyond the numbers on the scale, so pay attention to non-scale victories like increased energy, improved sleep, or better mental clarity.

5. Overcoming Plateaus and Challenges

Plateaus and challenges are common on any weight loss or lifestyle journey. When faced with a stall in progress or other obstacles, it's important to stay patient and proactive.

Strategies for Overcoming Plateaus

If you hit a weight loss plateau, consider adjusting your macronutrient ratios, increasing your physical activity level, or incorporating intermittent fasting. Experiment with different approaches to jumpstart your progress. Remember that weight loss is not always linear, and your body may be undergoing other positive changes even if the scale isn't moving.

Seeking Support and Accountability

Having a support system can greatly enhance your success and provide motivation during challenging times. Join online keto communities, find a workout buddy, or consider working with a registered dietitian or keto coach who can provide guidance, support, and accountability on your journey.

6. Long-Term Health Benefits of Keto

One of the significant advantages of adopting a ketogenic lifestyle is the potential for long-term health benefits beyond weight loss.

Improved Blood Sugar Control

A ketogenic diet can have a positive impact on blood sugar levels and insulin sensitivity. By minimizing carbohydrate intake and stabilizing blood glucose levels, a keto diet may help manage or prevent conditions like type 2 diabetes.

Reduced Inflammation

Inflammation is a root cause of many chronic diseases. The anti-inflammatory effects of the ketogenic diet, combined with the consumption of nutrient-dense foods, can help reduce inflammation in the body, potentially leading to improved overall health and a lower risk of diseases such as heart disease, cancer, and autoimmune disorders.

Enhanced Cognitive Function

Ketones, the byproduct of fat metabolism in a ketogenic state, are known to be an excellent fuel source for the brain. Many individuals report improved mental clarity, focus, and cognitive function while following a keto diet. This may have long-term implications for brain health and reducing the risk of cognitive decline.

7. Embracing a Whole-Food Approach

While it's possible to follow a ketogenic diet using processed low-carb products, adopting a whole-food approach is key to long-term sustainability and optimal health.

Benefits of a Whole-Food Approach

Whole foods are minimally processed and provide a wide range of nutrients, including vitamins, minerals, fiber, and phytochemicals. By prioritizing whole foods on your ketogenic diet, you can ensure you're nourishing your body with high-quality, nutrient-dense ingredients.

Focus on Nutrient Density

Include a variety of nutrient-dense foods in your meals, such as leafy green vegetables, cruciferous vegetables, lean proteins, healthy fats, and low-glycemic fruits. These foods provide essential vitamins, minerals, and antioxidants that support overall health and well-being.

Meal Planning and Preparation

Taking the time to plan and prepare your meals in advance can greatly contribute to the sustainability of your keto lifestyle. Set aside time each week to plan your meals, create a shopping list, and prepare ingredients or meals in advance. This will help you make healthier choices and avoid relying on convenient, but less nutritious options.

8. Practicing Mindful Eating

Incorporating mindful eating practices into your keto journey can enhance your overall relationship with food and support sustainable habits.

Benefits of Mindful Eating

Mindful eating involves paying attention to your eating experience, being present in the moment, and listening to your body's hunger and fullness cues. It helps promote a healthy mindset around food, prevents overeating, and fosters a deeper connection with the nourishment you provide your body.

Practicing Mindful Eating on Keto

Slow down and savor each bite, paying attention to the flavors, textures, and satisfaction you derive from your meals. Tune in to your body's hunger and fullness signals, eating until you feel comfortably satisfied, rather than overly full. Avoid distractions while eating, such as screens or multitasking, to fully engage in the experience of nourishing yourself.

9. Nurturing a Positive Mindset

Adopting a positive mindset is crucial for long-term success on your keto journey. Cultivating self-compassion, embracing the learning process, and reframing setbacks as opportunities for growth, can empower you to overcome challenges and maintain sustainability.

Self-Compassion and Self-Care

Be kind and patient with yourself throughout your keto journey. Celebrate your successes, no matter how small, and practice self-care to support your overall well-being. Engage in activities that bring you joy, reduce stress, and promote self-care, such as mindfulness practices, journaling, or engaging in hobbies.

Embracing the Learning Process

Approach your keto journey with a growth mindset, recognizing that it's a continual learning process. Be open to experimenting with new recipes, adjusting your approach, and discovering what works best for your body and lifestyle. Embrace the opportunity to learn more about nutrition, cooking, and yourself along the way.

Reframing Setbacks

Setbacks are a natural part of any lifestyle change. Instead of viewing setbacks as failures, reframe them as learning experiences and opportunities for growth. Reflect on what you can learn from setbacks and use them as stepping stones to propel you forward on your keto journey.

10. Seeking Professional Support

If you're facing challenges or struggling with the sustainability of your ketogenic lifestyle, seeking professional support can provide valuable guidance and motivation.

Registered Dietitian or Nutritionist

Consider working with a registered dietitian or nutritionist who specializes in ketogenic diets. They can provide personalized guidance, address any concerns or questions you may have, and help tailor your ketogenic approach to your individual needs and goals.

Healthcare Professional

Consult with your healthcare professional, especially if you have pre-existing health conditions or if you're making significant changes to your diet. They can provide insights, monitor your progress, and ensure that your ketogenic approach aligns with your overall health.

11. The Role of Community and Support

Building a supportive community can significantly contribute to the sustainability of your keto journey. Surrounding yourself with like-minded individuals who share similar goals and challenges can provide encouragement, accountability, and motivation.

Online Keto Communities

Joining online keto communities, forums, or social media groups can connect you with a vast network of individuals on similar journeys. These communities offer a space to share experiences, ask questions, seek advice, and celebrate milestones. Engaging with others who understand the unique aspects of a ketogenic lifestyle can foster a sense of belonging and provide valuable support.

Accountability Partners

Finding an accountability partner or workout buddy who is also following a ketogenic diet can be incredibly beneficial. You can check in with each other regularly, share progress, exchange meal ideas, and offer support during challenging times. Having someone to share the ups and downs of your journey can help you stay committed and motivated.

Family and Friends

Educating your family and friends about the ketogenic diet can foster understanding and support. Share your goals, explain the benefits, and provide resources or meal ideas that align with your dietary preferences. By involving your loved ones in your journey, you can create a supportive environment that makes it easier to sustain your keto lifestyle.

12. Mindful Eating Strategies for Long-Term Success

Developing mindful eating habits can support the sustainability of your keto lifestyle by promoting a healthy relationship with food and preventing overeating.

Eating with Awareness

Pay attention to your hunger and fullness cues. Eat when you're genuinely hungry, and stop eating when you feel comfortably satisfied, rather than aiming to clean your plate. Practicing mindful eating allows you to honor your body's signals and maintain a balanced approach to food.

Savoring the Flavors

Take the time to truly enjoy your meals. Slow down, chew your food thoroughly, and savor the flavors and textures. Engaging all your senses in the eating experience can enhance satisfaction and prevent mindless overeating.

Evaluating Emotional Hunger

Distinguish between physical hunger and emotional hunger. Emotional eating can lead to overconsumption and hinder your progress. When you feel the urge to eat, pause and ask yourself if you're truly hungry or if there's an emotional trigger at play. Find alternative ways to address emotions or stress, such as practicing self-care activities or seeking support from loved ones.

13. Honoring Your Body's Needs

Listening to your body and honoring its needs is crucial for long-term sustainability on a ketogenic diet.

Flexibility and Intuitive Eating

Allow for flexibility within the guidelines of the ketogenic diet. Tune in to your body's cravings and preferences, making adjustments when necessary. Intuitive eating involves trusting your body's wisdom and giving yourself permission to enjoy a variety of keto-friendly foods while staying mindful of your overall health goals.

Self-Care and Stress Management

Prioritize self-care and stress management to support your overall well-being. Engage in activities that bring you joy, promote relaxation, and reduce stress. This could include practicing mindfulness, engaging in regular exercise, spending time in nature, or pursuing hobbies that nourish your mind and body.

14. Long-Term Health Benefits of a Keto Lifestyle

Beyond weight loss, a ketogenic lifestyle offers numerous long-term health benefits that contribute to its sustainability.

Metabolic Health

A ketogenic diet can improve metabolic health markers, including blood sugar levels, insulin sensitivity, and blood lipid profiles. This can reduce the risk of metabolic disorders such as type 2 diabetes and metabolic syndrome.

Heart Health

The ketogenic diet may improve cardiovascular health by promoting weight loss, reducing inflammation, and improving blood pressure and cholesterol levels. These factors contribute to a lower risk of heart disease.

Brain Health

The brain benefits from ketones as an alternative fuel source. Ketones provide a stable and efficient energy supply, potentially enhancing cognitive function, focus, and mental clarity. This may have long-term implications for brain health and reducing the risk of age-related cognitive decline.

15. Embracing a Growth Mindset

Adopting a growth mindset is essential for long-term sustainability and adaptation on your keto journey.

Learning and Experimentation

Approach your keto lifestyle as a continuous learning experience. Be open to trying new recipes, experimenting with different approaches, and adapting your dietary choices based on your evolving needs and goals. Embrace the opportunity to expand your knowledge about nutrition and wellness.

Embracing Setbacks as Learning Opportunities

View setbacks or challenges as opportunities for growth and learning, rather than as failures. Understand that setbacks are a natural part of any lifestyle change and can provide valuable insights into areas where you can improve. Reframe setbacks as stepping stones to success and use them as motivation to continue moving forward.

16. Staying Motivated and Reinforcing Habits

Maintaining motivation is essential for long-term sustainability on your keto journey. Here are some strategies to stay motivated and reinforce positive habits:

Setting Meaningful Goals

Define specific and meaningful goals that go beyond just weight loss. Focus on goals such as improved energy levels, better mental clarity, or enhanced athletic performance. Having clear objectives will keep you motivated and provide a sense of purpose throughout your keto journey.

Tracking Progress

Regularly track your progress to monitor your success and stay motivated. Keep a record of your measurements, weight, body composition, and other relevant markers. Celebrate milestones along the way, no matter how small, to maintain a positive mindset and reinforce the progress you've made.

Rewarding Yourself

Create a system of rewards for achieving your goals. Treat yourself to non-food rewards such as a new workout outfit, a massage, or a weekend getaway. Celebrating your accomplishments will provide an extra boost of motivation and reinforce the positive habits you've established.

Establishing Supportive Habits

Developing supportive habits can greatly contribute to the sustainability of your keto lifestyle. Here are a few habits to consider:

Meal Planning: Set aside time each week to plan your meals and create a shopping list. Having a well-thought-out plan will make it easier to stick to your keto diet and avoid last-minute unhealthy choices.

Preparing Meals in Advance: Batch cooking or meal prepping can save time and make it convenient to stick to your keto diet. Prepare and portion meals ahead of time, so you always have keto-friendly options readily available.

Practicing Mindful Eating: Develop a habit of mindful eating by slowing down, savoring your meals, and paying attention to your body's hunger and fullness cues. This will help you develop a healthier relationship with food and prevent overeating.

Regular Exercise Routine: Establish a consistent exercise routine that complements your keto lifestyle. Find activities you enjoy and make exercise a non-negotiable part of your daily or weekly schedule.

17. Continuing Education and Research

Staying informed about the latest research and developments in the field of nutrition and ketogenic diets can help you adapt your approach and make informed decisions.

Read Books and Articles: Invest time in reading books, articles, and scientific studies related to the ketogenic diet. This will deepen your understanding and help you stay up-to-date with the latest information.

Attend Workshops and Webinars: Participate in workshops, webinars, or seminars led by experts in the field. These events offer opportunities to learn from knowledgeable professionals and engage in discussions with like-minded individuals.

Follow Trusted Sources: Follow reputable sources such as registered dietitians, nutritionists, and keto experts on social media or subscribe to their newsletters. These sources can provide valuable insights, tips, and updates on the keto lifestyle.

18. Embracing Flexibility and Evolving Needs

As your keto journey progresses, your needs and goals may evolve. Embracing flexibility and being open to adjusting your approach will contribute to the long-term sustainability of your keto lifestyle.

Periodic Assessments: Regularly assess your progress, goals, and dietary preferences. Determine if any modifications or adjustments need to be made to optimize your keto experience.

Trying New Recipes: Keep your keto meals interesting by exploring new recipes and experimenting with different ingredients and flavors. This will help you stay excited about your meals and prevent monotony.

Listening to Your Body: Tune in to your body's signals and adjust your dietary choices accordingly. If certain foods don't agree with you or if you're experiencing specific cravings, find alternative options that still align with your keto principles.

Conclusion

Sustainability and adaptation are key aspects of a successful long-term ketogenic lifestyle. Stay motivated, track your progress, establish supportive habits, and continue educating yourself about the keto diet. Embrace flexibility, reward yourself for achievements, and be open to evolving needs. By implementing these strategies, you can ensure the sustainability of your keto journey and enjoy the lasting benefits it offers for your health and well-being.

Chapter 11

Your Keto Lifestyle: Tips and Tricks for Success

In this final chapter, we will explore various tips and tricks to help you succeed in your keto lifestyle. These strategies will support your journey, provide practical guidance, and enhance your overall experience with the ketogenic diet.

1. Prioritize Whole, Nutrient-Dense Foods

Emphasizing whole, nutrient-dense foods is fundamental to a healthy and sustainable keto lifestyle. Here are some key considerations:

Fresh Vegetables: Make non-starchy vegetables the cornerstone of your meals. They provide essential vitamins, minerals, and fiber while adding flavor and variety to your dishes.

Quality Protein Sources: Opt for high-quality protein sources such as lean meats, poultry, fish, eggs, and plant-based proteins like tofu or tempeh. These foods help build and repair tissues, support muscle health, and contribute to satiety.

Healthy Fats: Incorporate healthy fats from sources like avocados, nuts, seeds, olive oil, coconut oil, and fatty fish. These fats provide energy, support brain health, and help you feel satisfied.

Limited Processed Foods: Minimize your consumption of processed foods, which often contain additives, preservatives, and hidden sugars. Choose whole foods whenever possible for optimal health benefits.

2. Meal Planning and Preparation

Meal planning and preparation are essential components of a successful keto lifestyle. By being organized and prepared, you can stay on track and minimize the chances of making impulsive, unhealthy choices. Here's how to approach meal planning and preparation:

Plan Ahead: Set aside time each week to plan your meals and create a shopping list. Consider your schedule, food preferences, and nutritional needs when designing your meal plan.

Batch Cooking: Dedicate a specific day or time to batch cook your meals for the week. Cook in larger quantities and portion out your meals for easy grab-and-go options.

Make Extra: When preparing meals, make extra portions that can be stored in the freezer for later use. This will save you time on busy days and prevent the temptation of ordering takeout.

Pre-Chop Ingredients: Prepare ingredients in advance by washing, chopping, and storing them in airtight containers. This will streamline your cooking process and make mealtime preparation more efficient.

3. Snacking and Keto-Friendly Options

Snacking can be a part of your keto lifestyle if done mindfully. Here are some tips for keto-friendly snacking:

Whole-Food Snacks: Choose whole foods as snacks, such as raw vegetables, nuts, seeds, olives, or cheese. These options provide nutrients and healthy fats while keeping your carbohydrate intake in check.

Portion Control: Be mindful of portion sizes, especially with calorie-dense snacks like nuts. Use small containers or portion out snacks in advance to avoid overeating.

Pre-Packaged Keto Snacks: There is an increasing availability of pre-packaged keto snacks on the market. While convenient, be mindful of their ingredients and nutritional profiles. Read labels carefully, as some products may contain hidden sugars or artificial additives.

4. Dining Out on Keto

Eating out doesn't have to derail your keto lifestyle. With some preparation and careful choices, you can enjoy restaurant meals while staying true to your dietary goals. Consider these strategies:

Research the Menu: Look up the restaurant's menu online before dining out. Identify keto-friendly options or dishes that can be easily modified to fit your needs.

Choose Protein-Based Dishes: Opt for protein-based dishes like grilled meats, seafood, or salads with protein. Request modifications, such as dressing on the side or extra vegetables instead of starches.

Be Mindful of Hidden Carbohydrates: Be aware of hidden carbohydrates in sauces, dressings, and condiments. Ask for them on the side or choose low-carb alternatives whenever possible.

Don't Be Afraid to Ask: Don't hesitate to communicate your dietary preferences to the server or chef. Most restaurants are willing to accommodate special requests or provide ingredient information to help you make informed choices.

5. Managing Social Situations

Navigating social situations can sometimes be challenging when following a keto lifestyle. However, with some preparation and communication, you can enjoy social events without compromising your dietary goals. Here are some strategies:

Communicate in Advance: If you're attending a social gathering, inform the host about your dietary preferences. Offer to bring a keto-friendly dish to share, ensuring there's something you can enjoy.

Focus on the Protein and Vegetables: At parties or events, focus on protein-rich foods and non-starchy vegetables. These options are often available and align well with your keto lifestyle.

Bring Keto-Friendly Snacks: If you're unsure about the food options available, bring your own keto-friendly snacks to ensure you have something to enjoy while socializing.

Practice Mindful Eating: Be mindful of your choices and portion sizes during social events. Take your time, savor each bite, and listen to your body's hunger and fullness cues.

6. Staying Hydrated

Proper hydration is important for overall health and well-being, especially on a ketogenic diet. Here are some tips to stay hydrated:

Water: Make water your primary beverage and aim to drink an adequate amount throughout the day. Carry a reusable water bottle with you as a reminder to stay hydrated.

Electrolyte Balance: The keto diet can affect electrolyte balance, so it's crucial to replenish essential minerals like sodium, potassium, and magnesium. Consider incorporating electrolyte-rich foods or using electrolyte supplements if necessary.

Herbal Teas and Infusions: Enjoy herbal teas or infuse water with fruits, herbs, or cucumbers for added flavor and hydration. Be cautious with fruit infusions as they may contain more carbohydrates.

7. Practicing Mindful Eating Habits

Mindful eating can enhance your relationship with food, support portion control, and improve overall satisfaction. Here are some mindful eating practices:

Slow Down: Take your time to chew each bite thoroughly and savor the flavors of your food. Eating slowly allows you to appreciate the experience and recognize satiety cues.

Pay Attention to Hunger and Fullness: Tune in to your body's hunger and fullness signals. Eat when you're physically hungry and stop eating when you're comfortably satisfied, rather than overly full.

Eliminate Distractions: Avoid distractions like screens, phones, or work while eating. Focus solely on the act of eating, allowing yourself to fully enjoy and engage with your meal.

Practice Gratitude: Before starting your meal, take a moment to express gratitude for the food you're about to eat. Cultivating gratitude can create a positive and mindful eating environment.

8. Implementing Intermittent Fasting

Intermittent fasting is a practice that involves alternating periods of fasting and eating. It can complement a ketogenic lifestyle and offer additional benefits. Here are a few popular intermittent fasting methods:

16/8 Method: This involves fasting for 16 hours and restricting your eating window to 8 hours. Typically, this is achieved by skipping breakfast and beginning to eat at noon, then finishing dinner by 8 p.m.

24-Hour Fast: This involves fasting for a full 24 hours once or twice a week. For example, you might eat dinner one evening and then not eat again until dinner the next day.

5:2 Diet: This approach involves eating normally for five days of the week and restricting calorie intake to around 500-600 calories on two non-consecutive days.

It's important to listen to your body and adapt intermittent fasting to your individual needs and lifestyle. Consult with a healthcare professional or registered dietitian if you have any concerns or specific health conditions.

9. Managing Keto Flu and Potential Side Effects

When transitioning to a ketogenic diet, some individuals may experience keto flu or other temporary side effects. Here are some strategies to manage these symptoms:

Adequate Hydration: Ensure you're drinking enough water and replenishing electrolytes to avoid dehydration and electrolyte imbalances that can contribute to keto flu symptoms.

Gradual Transition: Gradually reduce carbohydrate intake over a period of time rather than making abrupt changes. This can help minimize the severity of keto flu symptoms.

Increase Healthy Fats: Prioritize healthy fats in your meals to provide sustained energy and support the transition to a fat-burning state.

Supportive Supplements: Consider incorporating supplements such as electrolytes, omega-3 fatty acids, and magnesium to support overall health during the transition.

Remember that these symptoms are temporary and should subside as your body adapts to the ketogenic diet. If symptoms persist or are severe, consult with a healthcare professional.

10. Celebrating Non-Scale Victories

While weight loss may be a primary goal for many, it's important to celebrate non-scale victories as well. These victories include improvements in energy levels, mental clarity, sleep quality, and overall well-being. Acknowledge and appreciate the positive changes that extend beyond the numbers on the scale.

11. Staying Hydrated

Hydration is crucial for overall health and well-being, especially when following a ketogenic diet. Here are some tips to ensure you stay adequately hydrated:

Drink plenty of water: Make water your primary beverage and aim to consume at least eight glasses (64 ounces) of water per day. Carry a water bottle with you to stay hydrated on the go.

Monitor electrolyte balance: When following a ketogenic diet, your body may excrete more electrolytes, such as sodium, potassium, and magnesium. Ensure you're replenishing these electrolytes by including electrolyte-rich foods like leafy greens, avocados, nuts, and seeds in your meals. You can also consider adding an electrolyte supplement to your routine, especially if you're experiencing symptoms like muscle cramps or fatigue.

Enjoy herbal teas and infused water: Mix up your hydration routine by sipping on herbal teas or infusing your water with fruits, herbs, or cucumbers. This adds flavor and variety while keeping you hydrated throughout the day.

12. Prioritize Quality Sleep

Quality sleep is vital for overall health and plays a significant role in maintaining a successful keto lifestyle. Here are some tips to improve your sleep:

Establish a bedtime routine: Create a relaxing routine before bed to signal to your body that it's time to wind down. This can include activities like reading, taking a warm bath, practicing relaxation techniques, or listening to calming music.

Create a sleep-friendly environment: Ensure your sleep environment is cool, quiet, and dark. Use blackout curtains, earplugs, or a white noise machine if needed. Consider investing in a comfortable mattress, pillows, and breathable bedding to enhance your sleep quality.

Limit screen time before bed: Avoid using electronic devices, such as smartphones or tablets, before bed as the blue light emitted can disrupt your sleep-wake cycle. Instead, engage in activities that promote relaxation and prepare your mind and body for rest.

Maintain a consistent sleep schedule: Try to go to bed and wake up at the same time each day to regulate your body's internal clock. This helps establish a healthy sleep routine and promotes better sleep quality.

13. Practice Stress Management

Stress management is crucial for maintaining overall well-being and supporting your keto lifestyle. Here are some effective stress management techniques:

Exercise regularly: Engage in regular physical activity, such as walking, jogging, yoga, or strength training. Exercise helps reduce stress, improve mood, and boost overall well-being.

Practice relaxation techniques: Explore relaxation techniques such as deep breathing exercises, meditation, mindfulness, or progressive muscle relaxation. These techniques can help reduce stress, promote calmness, and enhance mental clarity.

Prioritize self-care: Make time for activities that bring you joy and relaxation. This can include hobbies, spending time in nature, practicing gratitude, journaling, or engaging in creative pursuits.

Seek support: Lean on your support system, whether it's family, friends, or a support group. Sharing your concerns and seeking guidance from others can help alleviate stress and provide a fresh perspective on challenges.

14. Celebrate Non-Scale Victories

In addition to tracking your progress based on the numbers on the scale, it's important to celebrate non-scale victories along your keto journey. Here are some non-scale victories to acknowledge and celebrate:

Increased energy levels: Notice how your energy levels have improved since starting the ketogenic diet. Celebrate the fact that you can now tackle daily activities with greater enthusiasm and vitality.

Improved mental clarity: Take note of how your mental clarity and focus have sharpened. Celebrate the enhanced cognitive function that allows you to think clearly and stay focused throughout the day.

Clothes fitting better: Pay attention to how your clothes fit and how your body shape may have changed. Celebrate the fact that you're making progress towards your goals and feeling more confident in your appearance.

Positive health markers: Celebrate improvements in health markers such as blood pressure, cholesterol levels, blood sugar control, or reduced inflammation. These improvements indicate that your body is responding well to the ketogenic diet.

15. Embrace the Journey and Stay Consistent

Remember that adopting a keto lifestyle is a journey, and it's essential to embrace it and stay consistent. Here are some final tips to help you on your path:

Be patient: Results may not happen overnight. Understand that sustainable changes take time, and consistency is key. Embrace the process and focus on long-term progress rather than immediate results.

Learn from setbacks: Setbacks are a natural part of any lifestyle change. If you experience a setback or slip-up, use it as an opportunity to learn and grow. Reflect on what led to the setback and adjust your approach moving forward.

Seek support: Surround yourself with a supportive community or find an accountability partner who shares your goals. Having someone to lean on, share experiences with, and seek guidance from can make your journey more enjoyable and successful.

Keep learning: Stay curious and continue learning about the ketogenic diet, nutrition, and health-related topics. This will help you stay informed, make informed choices, and adapt your approach as needed

16. Boosting Nutrient Intake

While the keto diet can be nutrient-dense, it's important to ensure you're getting a variety of essential vitamins and minerals. Consider the following tips to boost your nutrient intake:

Incorporate a variety of vegetables: Aim to include a diverse range of vegetables in your meals to maximize nutrient intake. Different vegetables offer unique profiles of vitamins, minerals, and antioxidants.

Choose quality protein sources: Opt for high-quality protein sources such as grass-fed beef, wild-caught fish, pasture-raised poultry, and organic eggs. These protein sources tend to contain more beneficial nutrients compared to conventionally raised options.

Include healthy fats: Consume a variety of healthy fats like avocados, olives, nuts, seeds, and cold-pressed oils. These fats provide essential fatty acids and fat-soluble vitamins.

Consider supplementation: Consult with a healthcare professional or registered dietitian to determine if supplementation is necessary to meet your nutritional needs. Common supplements on the keto diet include omega-3 fatty acids, vitamin D, and magnesium.

17. Maintaining a Healthy Mindset

A healthy mindset is vital for long-term success on your keto journey. Consider the following strategies to maintain a positive and sustainable mindset:

Practice self-compassion: Be kind to yourself and embrace self-compassion. Remember that the keto lifestyle is a journey, and it's natural to experience ups and downs along the way. Treat yourself with kindness and understanding.

Focus on non-scale victories: Celebrate achievements beyond the numbers on the scale. Notice improvements in energy levels, mental clarity, sleep quality, and overall well-being. These victories are equally important markers of success.

Surround yourself with support: Seek out a supportive community of like-minded individuals who can offer guidance, encouragement, and motivation. Share your experiences, challenges, and successes with others on a similar journey.

Embrace flexibility and balance: While the keto diet provides guidelines, it's important to find a balance that works for you. Allow yourself flexibility in your food choices and adapt the diet to fit your lifestyle and preferences.

Conclusion

Congratulations on completing this comprehensive guide to your keto lifestyle! By incorporating the tips and tricks discussed in this chapter, you'll be well-equipped to achieve long-term success on your keto journey. Prioritize gut health, track and adjust your approach as needed, incorporate intermittent fasting mindfully, boost nutrient intake, and maintain a healthy mindset. Remember that the keto lifestyle is a personal journey, and it's essential to listen to your body, make informed choices, and find what works best for you.

Closing Remarks

In conclusion, "The Ketogenic Diet Book for Beginners: Guide for Keto Lifestyle with Ease" has provided you with a comprehensive understanding of the ketogenic diet, its principles, and practical tips for successful implementation. Throughout this book, we have explored the science behind keto, essential kitchen setup, grocery shopping, cooking techniques, delicious recipes, overcoming challenges, incorporating exercise, sustainability, and adaptation, as well as tips and tricks for a successful keto lifestyle.

As you embark on your keto journey, remember that it is a lifestyle rather than a short-term solution. Embrace the process, stay committed to your goals, and be patient with yourself as you adapt to this new way of eating. The ketogenic diet offers numerous benefits, including weight loss, improved energy levels, mental clarity, and enhanced overall well-being.

Remember to listen to your body, make adjustments as needed, and seek support from a healthcare professional or registered dietitian if you have any concerns or specific health conditions. Stay curious, continue learning, and explore new keto-friendly foods, recipes, and techniques to keep your journey exciting and enjoyable.

May this book serve as a valuable resource and guide as you navigate the world of keto. Here's to your health, success, and a thriving keto lifestyle filled with delicious meals, newfound energy, and a renewed sense of vitality. Cheers to your keto journey!